COMMUNITY HEALTH NEEDS IN SOUTH AFRICA

The Making of Modern Africa

Series Editors: Abebe Zegeye and John Higginson

Community Health Needs in South Africa

NTOMBENHLE PROTASIA KHOTI TORKINGTON
Director of The Applied Research Centre and
Executive Dean of Hope in the Community,
Liverpool Hope University College

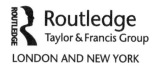

Routledge
Taylor & Francis Group

LONDON AND NEW YORK

First published 2000 by Ashgate Publishing

Reissued 2018 by Routledge
2 Park Square, Milton Park, Abingdon, Oxon OX14 4RN
711 Third Avenue, New York, NY 10017, USA

Routledge is an imprint of the Taylor & Francis Group, an informa business

A Library of Congress record exists under LC control number: 00132591

ISBN 13: 978-1-138-71627-8 (hbk)
ISBN 13: 978-1-138-71626-1 (pbk)
ISBN 13: 978-1-315-19713-5 (ebk)

Contents

List of Figures and Tables

Preface

Three weeks before I left for South Africa to undertake this research a friend came to wish me a good and fruitful sabbatical. She asked me a question which enabled me to voice the deep fears and anxieties I had had since it became evident that I was going to take a year off to conduct research on the health needs of black people in South Africa:

> Last summer I cycled from John O'Groats in Scotland to Land's End in Cornwall. I have always wanted to do this. It has been my lifelong ambition. Before I began my journey all my friends were saying how wonderful and exciting it was going to be and how brave I was to undertake such a journey. I shared in the feelings of excitement they had for me, but deep down there was the anxiety and the fear of moving from the known to the unknown. I remained anxious even when my friends in different parts of the country told me that they were going to come and spend some time with me when I cycled past their localities. What about you, how do you really feel about this project?

I admitted that underneath all the excitement and the anticipation of doing something I have always wanted to do, there was fear and anxiety. A number of factors contributed to my unease. South Africa is my home country and in that sense I was not going to a totally unknown situation. I knew for example, that I would not have major language difficulties, as I am fluent in two African languages and can understand and can make a good attempt at speaking a third. I am familiar with the norms and values that permeate black culture irrespective of where one is in South Africa. My first anxiety was around accommodation. I chose to have a base in the University of Cape Town rather than in a Durban University, closer to my family. Two reasons were influential in my decision. One was that I have always wanted to visit Cape Town but had not been able to do so whilst I lived in South Africa. Secondly, I wanted to be far enough from my family to ensure that the temptation to see the sabbatical as a year's holiday was minimised. I reasoned that a two-hour flight from Cape Town to Durban was a sufficient barrier in terms of both time and expense. Nevertheless, however valid these reasons might have been, I began to question my decision when four weeks before I was due to leave I had no accommodation arranged in Cape Town. The University offered me all academic facilities but no living quarters were available. My attempts to find a place to live by phoning estate agencies in Cape Town were not fruitful. This left me with a lot of anxiety.

The second anxiety was about the research itself. When asked to do a piece of research, it is usually well defined in terms of scope and parameters. It is true that in the life of a project one might be drawn into areas beyond the initial boundaries because of issues that emerge in the course of the research process, but in general, the boundaries are quite clear in the beginning in terms of the geographical area, the groups of people to be involved in the study and the methodologies to employ in the investigation. With a country as big as South Africa, and a topic as wide as health needs, anxiety is inevitable. I was excited about the opportunity to do the work but I also found the whole thing daunting. Where do I start? Will I be able to do it? Will people want to talk to me about their experiences? If they do, how will the research benefit them?

A year later, I was able to report I need not have had all those anxieties and fears, and for that I have a lot of people to thank. My accommodation problem was resolved three days before I flew to Cape Town. A close friend rang to inform me that she had not only found a place for me but that she was flying from Durban to Cape Town and with my landlady, was going to meet me at the airport.

Many other people contributed in different ways to make my sabbatical in South Africa enjoyable and fruitful. I wish to express my heartfelt gratitude to them all. I also want to explain that if some of the names do not appear in the acknowledgement it is not because I do not value their support and help, but if every name was included there would be no space left to write anything else. Also, my use of the pronoun 'we' in some areas reflects the strength of my feeling that this was a collective rather than an individual project. I would like, however, to mention a few people who played a critical role in reducing anxiety levels. I would like to thank Jane Moores who commissioned the research, for having enough trust in me to do the work. My many thanks to Professor Simon Lee, Rector and Chief Executive in Liverpool Hope University College, who trusted my ability to carry out the research and allowed me to have a year's sabbatical. My year's absence meant that my colleagues had to subsume my duties under their already heavy workload. I thank them all. In particular, I want to thank Martin Carey, my Co-Dean, in the Deanery of Hope in the Community.

Although my base was in Cape Town, in the course of the year I travelled to different parts of the country in order to get as broad a picture as possible of the health needs of black people. In the areas in which I worked I was fortunate enough to have families who kindly offered me accommodation. The people with whom I stayed provided me not only with their friendship but also took on the role of research assistants. They introduced me to people I needed to interview in their localities or professions and also provided the transport and on many occasions, stayed with me during the interviews. In Cape Town I wish to thank Joan Campbell in Durban, Dudu Malahleha and her husband, Dr Tohlang Malahleha, in Portshepstone, Thoko Somtyele, in Vulamehlo, Mangidi Mayeza and in Soweto, Maggie Mokgata. Without the friendship and the hospitality of these people my year in South Africa would not have been as pleasant as it was.

My sincere thanks also go to people who contributed substantially to the chapters included in the book. My thanks to Maggie Mokgata, Winnie Serobe and the Ikageng Women, Khathaso Mokoetle, Olga Lutu and the Women's Voice of Orange Farm, Molly Bailey and the Siyaphana women, Sr. Casian and the Women's Weaving Group, Mantombi Ngcobo, Thandeka Simoko, Florence Bhunu, Busi Nyembezi, Mabongi Mtshali, Mapula Chakane, Nonhlanhla Sokhulu, Thandazile Nhleko, Mabuyi Mnguni, Buyi Ngesi, Jabu Shezi, Dr Sebolelo Seape, Lauren Muller, Kathy De Filippi, Mrs Mooi, Peter Buckland, Graham Louw, Mark Kalil, Nomfundo Walaza, Petti Anderson, Lucy Nhlapo, Dr Tsakane Mpenyane, Sandra Brauda, Cosmas Desmond, Elsie Cliff, Chris Cody, Steve Smith, Dr Derek Timmins Nigel Mellor and Peter Davies. In addition there are people who gave me information and preferred to be identified as officers in their organisations. These include the Philani Nutrition Centre, St Luke's Hospice, Alexander Health Centre and University Clinic, Cancer Association of South Africa, Empilweni Community Mental Health Project and the Tsoga Environmental Project. To all these people I give my deepest thanks. I specifically want to thank the staff in Dr Mpenyane's surgery who distributed and collected the questionnaires and Mokobo Bushy Malahleha who helped with a similar task in the KwaZulu-Natal study.

It was the prompt and positive response from Professor Ken Jubber in the Department of Sociology, University of Cape Town, which encouraged me to pursue further the possibility of a year's sabbatical in South Africa. I would like to thank Ken and his colleagues very much for their hospitality and support. I would like to extend my thanks to the Library staff for their efficiency and their willingness to take me through their library system.

During my stay in South Africa I became friendly with a number of people outside the work situation. This enhanced my positive experience in the course of the study. In this category I would like to thank Zimitri Erasmus and Mary Simons.

Before my South African sabbatical I was computer illiterate. For the ability to use the laptop my gratitude extends to Toby Moores, Kevin Moores and Pat Kemble. Pat remained my e-mail link for advice when the computer refused to follow what it considered illogical commands.

My thanks to Loraine Gardner and Ian Vandewalle for the initial proof reading. I am indebted to Margaret Flynn for her excellent proof reading and editing skills. This book would never have materialised without Barbara Davies. Barbara has unmatched computer skills and patience. She spent countless hours with a computer which constantly 'froze' at the most critical moments. I am deeply indebted to Barbara, not only for her computer skills but also for her invaluable comments and suggestions.

A big thank you to my grand-daughters, Olivia Khoti and Chloe Nomakhosi Torkington and their parents Simon and Madeline for their support and understanding when planned weekends had to be cancelled in order to meet deadlines. Finally, I thank the black people in South Africa who spent so much of their time discussing their health needs with me.

Introduction

This book is the result of a study set up to investigate the health needs of black people in South Africa. The commission of the study was purposeful: to enable the identification of localities in which to make effective contributions to the development of competent health services. This was crucial in deciding the approach and the methodologies employed.

The epigram 'to understand the present and be able to plan for the future, we must know the past', is of particular relevance in South Africa. It is impossible to appreciate the present health needs of black South Africans without an understanding of the social, economic and political past which determined and shaped them. We look at that history in chapter one drawing from the work of theorists and their understanding of the factors that determined the way the South African social, political and economic structure evolved. The consequence of these for the health service is discussed in chapter two. In chapter three the focus is on the structure of the present health system.

Making a decision as to which dimensions of health care are to be included is not an easy task. It was made more difficult because of the methodologies adopted which were characterised by qualitative and participative ways of working. Ideas arising from in-depth interviews with individuals and representatives of organisations were embraced and feature in this text if they had something to add to our understanding of the health impacts of age and gender. The rationale is threefold. In any society that is based on inequalities, women, children and elderly people bear the brunt of these. Further, the future of any society is dependent on women and children. It is acknowledged that an individual's life chances are determined pre-natally by the health status of the mother. This suggests that the investment in children for the future has to start with ensuring that women are in good health, before and during pregnancy. The third is that in South Africa it has been women who have taken on board health related issues before and during the apartheid regime. It has been important from that point of view to see if under the African National Congress (ANC)

Government, the role of women in this area has changed, and to what effect.

Chapter four considers children and health, concentrating on the topics of malnutrition and violence. These feature prominently in the lives of black children and necessarily have created a lot of concern, not just for the present but for the future, since they cripple society at its roots. Chapter five on women and health focuses on the subjects of poverty, violence, prostitution and AIDS, all of which have implications for the health of women and future generations.

Under the apartheid system black women were subjected to triple oppression as capitalist, patriarchal and racial factors combined to subjugate them. Black women in different parts of the country are using the experience as a stepping stone to ensure that their families and communities survive well into the future. The different activities involved in this process are discussed in chapter six which is appropriately titled Women Making 'Herstory'. However, there is no suggestion here that women are overcoming all the problems. The point is that black women in South Africa are taking lead initiatives and are being very creative in the ways they problem-solve with their children and their communities in general. Chapter seven focuses on the experiences of elderly people and mental illness is the subject of chapter eight. Available statistics indicate that a large percentage of the black population, particularly the young, will be wiped out by AIDS. Issues around HIV/AIDS are discussed in chapter nine. While HIV/AIDS and mental illness have been included for the high profile they have, care for terminally ill people, the subject of chapter ten has a low public profile. Few people were aware of the invaluable work of hospices. Terminal care appears invisible to public gaze and consciousness for two reasons. Firstly, the medical model of health has subtly informed us that the dying are beyond help and therefore less resources need to be spent on them. Secondly, the dying are typically confined to the privacy of their families with very little help from outside the family circle. Thus, dying from a terminal illness, unlike accidental death, tends to be seen as an individual and private matter. My own understanding of death and dying in South Africa was nurtured by visits to the hospice centres in the three provinces - Western Cape, KwaZulu-Natal and Gauteng.

Chapter 11 reports on the results of a focus group discussion held in Orange Farm, an informal settlement in the Gauteng province.

Most of the chapters draw on qualitative data. In the process of conducting in-depth interviews some themes emerged which needed to be tested on a wider sample using questionnaires. Chapter 12 focuses on this quantitative data.

At the beginning of this book, action research as a philosophical approach is explored. My expectation of the 'action' component has been influenced by work experiences in Liverpool where the research process contributed to the setting up of tangible structures such as the centre for inherited blood disorders (Torkington, 1983), Mary Seacole House, a drop-in centre for black people with mental health problems, the Mental Health Black Advocacy Project, (Torkington, 1991), and the Translation and Interpreting Service (Mellor *et al*, 1990). These are tangible, pragmatic and very rewarding results which have made a difference in some people's lives. In South Africa the enormity of need can appear overwhelming and Chapter 13 considers ways in which a difference can be made against a backdrop of persistent poverty.

The chapters are preceded by a Submission to the Truth and Reconciliation Commission which will set the scene for the findings presented in the research.

Background to the Study

There are two main factors which led to my engagement with this study. One is my background and the other is Jane's relationship with South Africa. It is important at this stage to say something about these two factors because they have, and will continue to affect and inform the action research process in its various phases of development.

My Background

I was born and brought up in South Africa in a rural area on the South Coast of KwaZulu-Natal. I trained as a general nurse in the Eastern Cape and as a midwife in KwaZulu-Natal where I remained working in hospitals and clinics. The clinic served a large rural area. In addition to a structural base we also had a mobile, outreach component through which we met most of the users in designated stations - along dirt roads, in local churches, schools and grocery shops as well as in people's own homes. Although I had always been aware of the effects of apartheid on the health of black people, it was only when I worked in the health service that I realised just how devastating the impact was and how it permeated the whole of people's existence.

When South Africa was still in the grip of the apartheid system I came to England to pursue my studies in nursing after which I worked in general and children's hospitals. In England I have worked, and continue to work, on health issues with community groups, organisations in the public, private and voluntary sectors as well as with individuals. The approach I have adopted has been guided by the humane principles embodied in action research. Through these my understanding of health issues in general and more specifically, in relation to black people, has widened and deepened. It had been my long-held hope that when the opportunity arose, I would go to South Africa and contribute to a process that would play an unknown part in limiting and eventually eliminating the devastating situations I have lived and worked with and recently witnessed.

Jane's Background

Jane has had a long-standing relationship with South Africa and has contributed to various projects that provided badly needed services not available under the apartheid regime. With the liberation of the country in 1994 she sought to advance the development of the health service which, historically had so poorly served black people. Her knowledge of the health service is based on the experiences of friends and their relatives who had been subjected to appalling conditions in the public sector. She wanted to make a contribution that would be practical and realistic in terms of what could be achieved, given the available resources in relation to the health needs at both macro and micro levels. It was understood, for example, that providing needed housing, sanitation, water, fuel and employment, all very crucial elements in promoting good health, were not realistic goals in the short term. Neither was the building of hospitals that would demand huge capital and revenue investment. However, Jane also recognised the fact that advances were only possible if they were anchored within a wider understanding of South Africa's health system as perceived and experienced by service users and providers at grass-root level. This wider picture might enable other funders with an interest in facilitating the development of health services in South Africa, to see where their intervention might have the greatest impact. Thus, she commissioned the research.

Approaches and Methods

In undertaking this project the philosophical principles embodied in action research have been employed. To understand the guiding principles, the concept of action research will be explored before presenting the different methods used.

Action Research

Unlike the early 1950s, when the social sciences were dominated by a paradigm which stressed objectivity and value freedom, today most social scientists know and accept the validity of action research even if they themselves do not apply it in their work. Yet, like any other concept, the understanding of what action research means is as varied as the people who define it. For that reason it is important to clarify what I mean by action research. I start with a definition offered by early practitioners:

> ... a process whereby in a given problem area research is undertaken to specify the dimensions of the problem in its particular context; on the basis of this evidence, a possible solution is formulated and is translated into action with a view to solving the problem; research is then used to evaluate the action taken. In this way action research may appear to be challenging the application of social science to the solution of social problems by combining the knowledge and research techniques of social science both to discover solutions and to provide scientific evidence of their efficacy (Town, 1978, p.161).

This was the approach used to improve relationships between workers on the shop floor and management, with an expected increase in production. In the 1960s and early 1970s the approach was used in the analysis of social problems and in policy formation and implementation in Britain and the United States. Projects such as Education Priority Areas in the field of community development were guided by the principles of action research. These developments were in general welcomed by a discipline that had gained itself:

> ... the dubious 'smash and grab' image of research where researchers study a situation for their own purpose and depart with the vague promise that all will be revealed when the research report is finally published (Town, p.166).

Later, advocates for action research expressed a concern over the distinction that existed between 'research' as the domain of academics and 'action' as a field for activists and providers. They argued that such a division creates problems which include poor co-ordination, conflict of interest and a failure of action research to consider the political context and implications of a programme of action. To overcome these problems the scientists suggested the abandonment of any formal division between research and action responsibilities so that there is no institutionalised differentiation between the researcher or research team and the activists or action team (Ben Tovim et al, 1985).

The essence in what is being advocated above is that the researcher/research team and the research process must make a difference in the lives of people amongst whom research is conducted. This is only possible if the researchers become part of the process that seeks to bring about a positive change not only at the level of collecting statistics but also of following through by joining in the action which will bring about that change. It was from this understanding that I formulated a definition of action research which is operative in this study:

> Mainly action research is not about collecting statistics and compiling them for publications which are then claimed by the researcher for presentation at academic conferences. This is not to say that the collection of statistics and the production of publications or indeed participation in academic discourse is excluded or prohibited. But these are not the main objectives. The role of the researcher is to investigate issues affecting the community and using the results of that investigation, to work towards changing or influencing policies in order to redress the balance. This process cannot be set in motion unless researchers work with the communities affected by the existing policies and practices, as well as with organisations with the responsibility to meet the needs of the community (Torkington, 1991, p.163).

This must be the objective. Whether or not the researcher achieves it, and to what degree, is another matter. The important thing is that at the very beginning when the research area is chosen, and in the process of research itself, this must be the guiding principle - to make a difference in people's lives. That objective stands a better chance of being achieved if flexible techniques are used in collecting the methodology.

Methodology

In the process of gathering information I allowed a flexible, open and multi-dimensional approach which roughly falls under four headings – use of the existing literature, living with people, in-depth interviews and questionnaires.

Use of Existing Literature

Although I worked in the health service in South Africa, this was a long time ago and so many changes have taken place since then. But this in fact was an advantage because it forced me to approach the study with an open mind prepared to read material on health and related areas, ask questions, and listen before drawing conclusions and making recommendations. This engagement with the literature continued right through the investigation but it was more intensive in the University of Cape Town, the academic base which offered me access to library material.

Living with People

Books and journals written by informed theorists, researchers and activists are a very good source of information on the experiences of people, but these are no substitute for the contribution which comes from those who go through the experience. Not only can people identify their own needs but they can also suggest how those needs can be met. To access that information I lived with people and listened to what they said in their homes, churches, bible study groups, weddings, christenings, funerals, dinner parties, restaurants, universities, conferences, workshops, seminars, hospitals, clinics, surgeries and many other places. Getting information through living with people has a number of advantages.

The first is that people are not telling you as a researcher what happened or happens to them or to people they know. They are exchanging information as friends at a dinner party, as professionals in a workshop or as women coming to a women's centre with a variety of problems. They know that you are a researcher, as indeed for ethical reasons, this must be made clear from the outset, yet this is not uppermost in their minds when they talk about a specific incident or issue. The researcher simply becomes part of the group.

The second advantage is the opportunity to pursue themes which emerge with more than just one person. One or two questions asked without waving the research flag can change a dinner party into a workshop where people do not only talk about what has happened, but debate on what are the causes of those incidences and how they can be resolved. It is at these gatherings that I learned about child sexual abuse, the abuse of elderly people, violence against women, the effect of HIV/AIDS on individuals/families and many more. It is not only the information that is important but also an opportunity to find out what people feel are the real issues to be addressed and by whom and in what order of priority.

The third is that the groups provided an opportunity to meet people or to be informed of people who had more information on any of the issues discussed. This was partly how I compiled the list of people with whom I conducted in-depth interviews. A snowball effect came into operation as one interviewee referred me to others in the same or related fields. This network was invaluable, not only in meeting people who might not have agreed to be interviewed had I not been referred by those they knew, but also in creating a positive climate within which the interviews took place. The fact that I had been introduced by their colleagues or friends minimised the tension and lowered the barriers that characterised interviews I had with people who I approached outside of this network. There were of course exceptions where subtle barriers, such as tedious bureaucratic procedures before one is allowed to visit a hospital, remained intact irrespective of informal introductions. In these situations formal procedures were abandoned. Instead I moved from ward to ward looking for friends who were employees of the hospitals. In my search I had the opportunity to see the conditions under which people were treated. More importantly the network enabled me to cross-check certain details if there was conflicting information or a need for any clarification on any particular issue.

The final advantage in living with people as a research method is that one shares people's experiences as they live through them. When you have walked for miles with women and young girls to the river to fetch water and have taken over an hour to come back carrying a pail of water on your head, you get to know what that means to people who must do it four or five times a day. When that water is from a river which is not only a source of water for animals, which on occasion relieve themselves in it, not only a recipient of human excreta brought down by rains from slopes where people have no toilets, but also upstream is used as a laundering area for people's clothes, then you understand why people in that area get bouts of cholera which spreads like wildfire and kills hundreds of people.

When you go to where pensioners collect their pension and see hundreds of them sitting for hours in the heat, the cold or the rain, having left their homes before sunrise, and then after all that, for some to be told that their money is not showing on the computer, you get to know the financial plight of elderly people. They are only too aware that they are being swindled because the computer operator has just told them that next time they come a sum of so many Rands or so many chickens will enable the computer to find their names. They go home crying, having lost that month's pension with the prospect of losing more if they do not come with the Rands or the chickens. Even when they do, as one elderly person told us, it may take months before 'the computer' coughs up the money again. They know they are being robbed but they feel powerless and frightened to do anything about it. When people prop up dying elderly relatives and take them to collect their pension, you get to know what that pension means to the family. When you see a sick person being pushed in a wheelbarrow for miles before being able to get into a taxi which travels for at least 30 to 40 minutes before reaching a doctor's surgery, then you realise how inaccessible health services are for many people. In a taxi in which people are packed like sardines, and you are one of the sardines, you begin to understand why at high speed or in negotiating bends many taxis lose balance. You begin to understand why South Africa is the leading country in road traffic accidents. In all these situations there is little need for the spoken or written word since the researcher has access to the live experiences of people. What this sharing of experience does not give the researcher however, is how people perceive and interpret that experience and it is this that in-depth interviews attempt to elicit.

In-depth Interviews

This way of collecting information complemented or preceded the above methods. In a number of situations in which I 'lived' with people, themes were raised which needed to be followed up by in-depth interviews in order to get a deeper understanding of the issues involved. On the other hand in-depth interviews were conducted with people I met accidentally. The themes raised became a focal point for further exploration. My very first in-depth interview in Cape Town, for example, was with a young woman I met on a train. Before we parted she had told me about her original home in the rural areas, why she moved into Cape Town and what life was like in an informal settlement. It was this chance meeting which motivated me to visit informal settlements, not only in Cape Town but in other parts of the country. In this case the in-depth interview preceded and informed further research.

Although qualitative data encompasses issues that people raise as well as capturing perceptions and interpretations of those issues, it is nevertheless seen as insufficient as a basis for making meaningful generalisations. However, notions of generalisations become an issue if we believe that the situation becomes a reality only when it affects many people. If we start from the premise that even if one person is dehumanised in any way then something must be done to restore that person's dignity and humanity, the issue of numbers becomes irrelevant. I accept, however, that when it comes to providing a service, it is important that the views of as many people as possible are sought in order to determine that there is general agreement about what the issues are, what should be provided, and how it should be provided. It is in this context that the questionnaire method of collecting information was used in this research.

The Use of Questionnaires

Questionnaires were used as one of the many methods employed in data collection. The themes for the questionnaires came from discussions with different individuals and groups in the course of the research and from a workshop held in a surgery in Orange Farm, an informal settlement in Gauteng. I shall discuss in detail the problems associated with using this method of collecting information in the South African situation. Whatever the problems, the quantitative data, in conjunction with the rest of the information collected using other methods mentioned above, was very useful in giving the wider and deeper understanding of the South African health system. To put that understanding in context we need to provide a historical background of South African society and the development of health services within it.

Submission to the Truth and Reconciliation Commission Concerning Forced Removals

The United Nations' International Convention on the Suppression and Punishment of the Crime of Apartheid states:

> the term 'the crime of apartheid'... shall apply to the following inhuman acts committed for the purpose of establishing and maintaining domination by one racial group of persons over any other racial group of persons and systematically oppressing them:
>
> (b) Deliberate imposition on a racial group or groups of living conditions calculated to cause its or their physical destruction in whole or in part;
>
> (d) Any measures, including legislative measures, designed to divide the population along racial lines by the creation of separate reserves and ghettos for the members of a racial group
>
> (e) Exploitation of the labour of the members of a racial group

The Convention on the Prevention and Punishment of the Crime of Genocide states:

> In the present Convention, genocide means any of the following acts committed with intent to destroy, in whole or in part, a national, ethnical, racial or religious group, as such:
>
> (b) Causing serious bodily or mental harm to the group;
>
> (c) Deliberately inflicting on the group conditions of life calculated to bring about its physical destruction in whole or in part.

We submit that the systematic dispossession of the black population of South Africa – which started in 1652, reached its height in the last third of the nineteenth century, and which was ruthlessly pursued towards its logical, genocidal conclusion by the apartheid government – falls within the scope of both these Conventions. We will concentrate on the Nationalist government's policy of forced removals, though this policy can only be understood in the light of the history of colonialism.

As a 'crime against humanity' and a genocidal practice, we submit that this was clearly one of the most gross violations of the human rights of the vast majority of the population in south Africa one that is not being redressed by the Government of National Unity's land reform programme – consisting of land restitution, redistribution, and tenure reform – which will benefit only a minority of the dispossessed.

The Land Restitution Act will only benefit those who were removed from land to which they held legal title, of whom there were relatively few. In any event, most of them did receive alternative, albeit often inferior, land, even if their original land is restored to them this will add only an infinitesimal amount of land to the total owned by Africans. Land redistribution will be a very slow and partial process. The present objective is to redistribute 18.5 percent of the land by 2007, which the government estimates will satisfy only 56 percent of land hunger. The Tenure Reform programme will largely benefit labour tenants and farm workers, but will do little, if anything, for the 1.2 million who were removed between 1960 and 1982.

There are, therefore, millions of people who were forcibly removed from land which they had occupied for generations for whom no provision is being made. These people not only lost their place of residence, and often their means of livelihood, many also lost all their possessions. Not only were they subjected to severe ill-treatment, which often resulted in death, particularly of children and old people, but they are still suffering from the impoverishment inflicted upon them.

We also suggest that the forced removal of people – sometimes at gun-point, often by threat of legal action, usually by the simple exercise of *force majeur* – from their home to a place not of their choosing, and from which there was no escape, constitutes 'abduction' and thus falls within the terms of reference of the Truth and Reconciliation Commission. There can be no doubt that people were *forcibly* removed, despite government claims that all removals were 'voluntary'. There are, for example, court records, as well as numerous eye-witness accounts.

While it is true that they were removed in accordance with the law, not only did those laws lack any moral foundation, they were also enacted by a government which it is now generally accepted was illegitimate. If apartheid never really existed, as we are now led to believe, then those laws did not exist either.

There can also be no doubt that the policy was politically motivated and that it necessarily and deliberately entailed 'severe ill-treatment' of people.

That ill-treatment was not due to the inefficiency of neglect of local officials. It was provided for in the regulations governing forced removals. In regard to 'closer settlements', for example, General Circular No 25 of 1967 states, 'normally only a rudimentary lay-out on the basis of agricultural residential areas is undertaken. A common source of water where the inhabitants can fetch their water. (No mention is made of from how far they might have to fetch it) is a prerequisite. The inhabitants are also expected to install their own cesspit latrines together with dwellings, traditional or otherwise'.

It is significant that, as far as we know, neither the regulations nor the statements of government spokesmen (there were no women) ever refer to those removed as 'people' they were 'Bantu', 'squatters', 'inhabitants', 'superfluous appendages', never people. If they were not people, there was no question of them having any rights.

The 'rudimentary lay-out' consisted of marking out 50 metre-square plots and providing a source of water, which was often a very muddy and shallow dam or a distant, and frequently dry, river: no schools, no clinics, no shops, no roads, no jobs, nothing. Some two million people who, by the government's own definition, consisted primarily of 'the aged, the unfit, widows, women with dependent children' were dumped in these conditions. Many did not survive, those who did are still the most impoverished people in the country. They were considered 'superfluous' then and they still are. There is no way in which they will ever be reintegrated into the economy through the workings of market forces. The Nationalist government went to great pains to get rid of them, at least equal pains must be taken to bring them back.

Attempts to forget about everything but the most brutal, individual excesses of apartheid do a great injustice to the millions of people who suffered under it and are still enduring its effects. Rarely, for example, does one meet an African family – particularly in the rural areas – that has not lost at least one child because of malnutrition or the lack of medical facilities, which were the direct result of the apartheid system, of which forced removals were a corner-stone.

Individuals *did* commit the most gross and inhuman crimes but it was apartheid itself that was a 'crime against humanity'. In both theory and practice it denied the humanity of the black population. And nowhere was this more evident than in its forced removal policy – euphemistically called 'resettlement' (the same euphemism that the Nazis used).

That policy did not only deny people's right to freedom of movement or their right to shelter, it deprived an unknown number of people of the most fundamental of rights, the right to life. People, particularly children and old people, died as a direct result of a deliberately implemented policy: a policy of which the National Party boasted Dr Piet Koornhof, who now claims that he was never responsible for any removals, stated in the House of Assembly on 4 February 1965, when he was Deputy Minister of Bantu Affairs:

> I want to ask how much progress we have made in respect of the implementation of that aspect of our policy, i.e. the elimination (sic) of the redundant, non-economically active Bantu in our white areas... approximately 900,000 Bantu have been settled elsewhere under the National Party regime over the past few years, since 1959. Surely this is no mean achievement; on the contrary, it is a tremendous achievement.

We further suggest that, while the responsibility for this gross violation of human rights rests primarily with office-bearers under the Nationalist government, others are also responsible. As the former Convention states: 'international criminal responsibility shall apply, *irrespective of the motive involved* (our emphasis) to individuals, members of organisations and institutions and representatives of the State... whenever they:

- commit, participate in, directly incite or conspire in the commission of the acts mentioned in Article II of the present Convention (see above);
- directly abet, encourage or co-operate in the commission of the crime of 'apartheid'.

Most white people did that; more especially those who exploited the cheap labour made available by the apartheid system. And none more so than the gold and diamond mining magnates who, as Kader Asmal and his co-authors have pointed out (*Reconciliation Through Truth*, David Philip, Cape Town, 1996), never questioned the morality of apartheid. Rather, 'they exploited the cruel migrant labour system and made unabashed use of apartheid labour, and actively peddled its availability as an advantage to international investors' (p.156). Misguided they might have considered apartheid to be; but it suited them. As Cyril Ramaphosa once remarked, 'it is the (mining) industry which provided the furnace in which racial discrimination was baked'.

We submit that they too should be called upon by the TRC to make reparation.

The migratory labour system was largely designed to meet their need for a plentiful supply of cheap labour. It was cheap because many of the costs were borne by their families who had been driven off the land and herded into 'reserves'. It was the women left behind to scrape some form of subsistence from a tiny piece of land who were responsible for the nurture, education, health, etc of the children, not the employers of their menfolk. Deprived of their land and forced, by laws passed at the instigation of the mining houses and others, to pay various taxes in cash, the men had no choice but to work for whatever pittance they were offered. For over a century the poorest people in the country have been subsidising the richest.

In particular, the migratory labour system led to the break up of families, which is probably the most important factor in the dramatic and alarming increase in the physical and sexual abuse of children. Those who benefited from that system, therefore, bear a direct responsibility for the many, very many, children who have been, and continue to be, abused. This responsibility cannot be discharged by allocating a minuscule percentage of post-tax profits to 'development'. The government's present provision for meeting the needs of these children is totally inadequate, because of budgetary constraints. Those who caused the problem should be obliged to help to solve it.

We are not concerned with apportioning blame or engendering guilt; but unless the full enormity of the evil is clearly exposed and recognised there is no possibility of people being prepared to make the necessary effort, even sacrifice, to compensate for it. If there was never any great problem, there is no need for any drastic solutions.

But there *was* a great problem, the ramifications of which are still not fully understood. As historian Colin Bundy writes, in relation to forced removals. 'What is still impossible to convey is the cumulative, collective, *epochal* character of the experience. None, yet, can convey the totality of the impact of social engineering under racial capitalism'.

We will give a brief overview and adduce some evidence to substantiate these suggestions, but we would also like to recommend that a number of publications, notably, *The Rise and Fall of the South African Peasantry*, by Colin Bundy, *Tomorrow's Sun*, by Helen Joseph. *The Discarded People*, by Cosmas Desmond, and *The Surplus People Project Reports* also be considered by the Commission as evidence of the heinousness of this crime.

The rape of one woman is a heinous crime, but we are talking about the rape of a whole nation, of which women and children were the main victims. We have accounts, for example, of heavily pregnant women being literally dumped in the middle of the barren veld with no shelter – let alone a bed – no medical facilities, often not even any water. Their labour induced by a bumpy ride on the back of a lorry, on arrival they gave birth – in the dust or the mud – to a baby whose chances of survival were virtually nil. What about their right to privacy, to medical care... to life?

In Limehill, one of the more publicised 'resettlement' areas, for example, there was, over the first ten years, an infant mortality rate of 22 percent (compared to about 1 percent for the white population), moreover, 11 percent of those aged under five, and perfectly healthy, at the time of the removal, did not survive those ten years. Further, the rate of population growth was halved. Was not that the purpose of the exercise? Is that not genocide? Children died not only like flies, but also covered with flies. We trust that at least some of the Commissioners will have endured the experience of seeing children die in this way and so will understand our concern and anger (Perhaps the Commission could organise a tourist trail to visit *their* graves rather than those of the 'fallen heroes' of the Boer War).

The history of forced removals, however, is not simply a multiplication of heart-rending stories of children dying from such diseases as typhoid and gastro-enteritis because of the lack of sanitation and a proper water supply. It is that and each instance was a tragedy for the family and the whole community, but it is also much more.

The forced removals policy was an attempt at social engineering on a scale not seen since Stalin. The 'ideal', as Dr Verwoerd said when he became Prime Minister, was 'total separation in all spheres'. The purpose, of such 'separate development', he stated in the House of Assembly on 4 April 1961, was to buy 'for the white man his freedom and the right to retain domination in what is his country'. No price was too high to pay – either in terms of the economy or, more importantly, in terms of peoples' lives – to achieve that end, which aimed at the total physical separation of blacks and whites in order to ensure the political subjugation and economic exploitation of the former.

The policy was based on the premise that Africans were 'labour units', not people: this implies a total denial of their human rights. As Dr Koornhof once explained:

> I am afraid to say that the... African males from the homelands have no rights whatsoever in South Africa. Their rights are in their own homelands, and they are in South Africa only to sell their labour.

It is impossible to put a figure on the number of people affected by this policy. It has been reliably documented that 3.5 million people were forcibly removed between 1960 and 1983, but many were removed before that date. Further, this figure does not include all those who were shunted around within the 'reserves' in the interests of so-called 'betterment schemes', nor the millions who found themselves deprived of their South African citizenship and transferred to an 'independent state' at the stroke of a pen, let alone the even more millions who were removed individually from the urban areas by being 'endorsed out'.

Nor does it include the relatively few, but very significant, yet totally forgotten people who were banished – at the whim of a Native Affairs Commissioner – to places hundreds, sometimes over a thousand, kilometres from their home and left to die there. These were the real leaders of the people who opposed the bantustan system from the outset, but who to-day has even heard of people like George Ramafoku, Paulus Mopeli, Maema Matlala, and many others?

There is no one simple explanation for all the varied forms of forced removals; the policy was continually adapted to meet the changing, and even conflicting, needs of the government's constituency – white farmers and the white working class – and the interests of capital. It was a part, an essential part, of the overall apartheid strategy of controlling every aspect of black people's lives in order to ensure the political supremacy and economic dominance of the white.

The suffering it caused goes far beyond 'severe ill-treatment'; the deaths are innumerable; its effects will be felt by people for generations. It was not a mistake, it was not a well-intentioned, but misguided, attempt to solve the 'native problem'. It was a well-planned and ruthlessly implemented policy which completely disregarded even the most fundamental rights of black people in order to preserve the privileges of whites. We believe, therefore, that it merits the most serious consideration by a Commission which is concerned with the 'gross violations of human rights'.

Probably most of those responsible for formulating and implementing this inhuman policy are now dead, but there is still the question of reparation.

As we have emphasised, this was not simply an exercise of mindless racism, the Nationalists knew what they were doing and why they were doing it, but they still did it. Nevertheless, the way in which it was done did owe much to the racism of the ruling class. It would not have been possible to inflict such conditions on anybody – let alone the aged, the infirm, the pregnant – if you believed that they bled as you did, that they were 'fed with the same food, hurt with the same weapons, subject to the same diseases'. Racist myths had, therefore, to be created to 'justify' Africans being treated as a sub-human species.

The whole party of apartheid, and of forced removals in particular, was based on the denial of the humanness of the African people. There cannot be a more gross violation of human rights than that.

Anybody who has seen the despair, the confusion, the powerlessness of people who had been summarily uprooted from their established homes and dumped in the veld cannot but be amazed that not only have many of them survived but they have actually managed to re-build some form of community. They have not accepted, but they have come to terms with their fate. This is a tribute to their resilience, courage, ingenuity, and the very humanness which was consistently denied by the apartheid regime.

They need, and deserve, recognition and recompense.

The attached testimonies do not refer to the worst cases which could be found even in such a limited area as the lower South Coast; they are rather randomly selected examples of the effects which such apartheid legislation as the Group Areas Act, the Prevention of Illegal Squatting Act, and the Land Acts had on the lives and the rights of ordinary people.

The people still bitterly remember the day they were forcibly removed and they remain impoverished because of their dispossession. They believe they have the right to reparation and to re-integration into the economic, social and political life of the country from which they have been deliberately excluded for decades.

In an African context, all talk of developing a human rights culture is meaningless if people who belong to the land do not have land to cultivate. Their relationship to the land is still, for the majority of South Africans, the basis of their culture. Before we can have a human rights culture, we have to have a culture. The whole land question, therefore, cannot be divorced from any discussion about human rights.

Forcibly to deprive people of their land is unquestionably a gross violation of their human rights. To do so on the scale that the apartheid regime did it is a crime so horrendous that the Truth and Reconciliation Commission, we submit, simply cannot ignore it. For millions of South Africans it is *the* human rights issue, which cannot be dealt with through the very slow and very limited land restitution process envisaged by the government's land reform programme.

At the very least, the heinousness of this crime must be publicly recognised by the Commission and some immediate reparation must be made (Presented by Desmond on behalf of a number of NGOs, 1997).

References

Ben-Tovim, G., Gabriel, J., Law, I. and Stredder, K. (1986), *The Local Politics of Race*, MacMillan.

Desmond, C. (1997), *The Truth and Reconciliation Commission*, presented by Desmond on behalf of a number of NGOs.

Mellor, N., Torkington, N.P.K. and Ben-Tovim, G. (1990), *A Translation and Interpreting Service for Merseyside*, Liverpool City Council.

Torkington, N.P.K. (1983), *The Racial Politics of Health – A Liverpool Profile*, Liverpool University.

Torkington, N.P.K. (1991), *Black Health – A Political Issue*, Catholic Association for Racial Justice and Liverpool Institute of Higher Education.

Town, S.W. (1978), 'Action Research and Social Policy: British Experience' in Bulmer, M. (ed), *Social Policy Research*, MacMillan.

Glossary

Afrikaner	Descendants of Dutch people who settled in South Africa in 1652
ANC	African National Congress
Bond	Mortgage
Coloured	People of mixed ethnic origin
Compound	Living accommodation for mine workers (hostel)
CHW	Community health worker
ECT	Electro-convulsive therapy
Homelands	Areas set aside by the Nationalist Government for occupation by black people
Informal Settlements	Settlements with no formal authorisation which have no services or infrastructure
Medical Aid Schemes	Private medical insurance
NCAW	National Council of African Women
NGO	Non-Governmental Organisation
NPPHCN	National Progressive Primary Health Care Network
Peri-Urban	Settlements near towns
PHC	Primary Health Care
RDP	Reconstruction and Development Programme
Shacks	Makeshift housing structures
South African rate of exchange	£1 = R10 ± (1999 rates)
Spaza Shops	Mobile shops
Street Committees	Committees set up by United Democratic Front in the 1980s to organise and maintain law and order in black townships
Township/Location	Densely populated settlement for black people separate from white living areas
TBA	Traditional birthing assistant
WHEP	Women's Health and Empowerment Programme

1 The Historical Development of South African Society

A doctor who genuinely wants to heal her patient will look beyond the physical symptoms, and examine everything in the patient's environment which is a likely cause of the symptoms. Similarly, the social analysis of diseases requires that we should examine the society to see which aspects of it are responsible for causing ill health, and then work for whatever changes are necessary and possible to improve the situation. This takes us out of the world of pure medicine and into that of politics - a necessary step. The barriers that have been erected between health and politics are artificial. They must be broken down before we can even begin to think what a healthy society might look like (De Beer, 1984).

As De Beer points out, it is important that we have some idea of the society within which South Africa's present health system developed in order to understand the enormous task faced by the government in its attempt to improve the health of the nation. Such understanding will also be useful for those who are interested in contributing to the development of good health for people in South Africa. They too need to know that current health issues have their roots in a history that predates the apartheid era. If good health is to be realised it matters that the focus is not only on illness and disease but also on the well-established roots that feed illness and disease.

Theoretical Perspectives in the Development of South African Social, Political and Economic Structure

The history of South Africa, which is relevant in explaining present patterns of disease and health care, has roots reaching back to 1652 when the first white settlers from the Netherlands landed in the Cape of Good Hope. From the time the settlers arrived contact between black and white people was characterised by wars over the possession of land and cattle.

1

As De Kiewiet (1950) points out however, this era was skewed by more than just the desire to have land. It was primarily a process which gave the white community more than the bulk of the best land. They gained a considerable measure of control over the labour power of black people. Black people lost access to their land and were only allowed to work on it as labourers, tenants or herdsmen.

The control of land was finally legalised by the Land Tenure Act of 1913 which gave 87 percent of the land to white people and 13 percent to black people. This disproportionate distribution of land, many analysts have argued, is the heart of all developments which have impacted negatively on the health of black people. To many, racism was the impetus for these developments, but others maintain that racism was less influential in pursuing its own interests than the pursuit of capital. One such theorist is Wolpe who traces these developments back to the early phases of capitalism.

Wolpe (1972) proposes that during the early phases of capitalist development, when extractive industries and agriculture were the main employers of labour, the rural economy subsidised capitalism by making it possible for the extended family to perform 'Social Security' functions for the reproduction of the migrant labour force. It was the work of the family to care for the young, the old, the sick and the migrant workers when they were not at work. Thus, rural black families were crucial for capitalism since it was through the network of reciprocal obligations between the migrant workers and their rural families that a system of cheap labour through migration was maintained. This rural 'subsidy' enabled the white employer to fix wages at persistently depressed levels to provide subsistence to the migrant workers and only during their period of actual employment. Wages were woefully inadequate to maintain labourers and their families.

By 1920 the pre-capitalist forms of production surviving in rural areas began to show signs of decline for a number of reasons, e.g. the absence of able-bodied migrants, the increasing pressure exerted by population expansion and the incapacity of rural land to increase agricultural production as a result of inefficient farming methods. Such factors made agricultural production so precarious that the slightest drought such as that which occurred between 1934 and 1936, could cause a serious deficit in the production of African staple foods, i.e. the production of maize dropped from 3.7 million bags in 1934 to 1.2 million in 1936 and sorghum production fell from 1.2 million bags to 0.5 million bags in the same period. Rural poverty prevailed and as a result many people left to seek work in the cities.

The period between 1940 and 1960 was characterised by diverse industrial and political conflicts which were met and suppressed by oppressive political measures which formed the nucleus of apartheid. These conflicts coincided with a rapid expansion in the secondary and tertiary sectors of industry most of which were owned by British capital or English speaking South Africans. Since these industries needed a larger skilled work force, more than that provided by the white working class, the owners sought to solve their employment problems, and at the same time resolve the conflicts, by relaxing the political and the economic constraints on black workers. However, this had to be done without a corresponding fall in profits, and since this could only be achieved by reducing the wages of white workers, most of whom were of Afrikaner stock, the Afrikaners opposed this solution and their feelings were reflected in the victory of the Nationalist Party in 1948. This heralded a comprehensive repression of black people. By protecting white workers from the competition of black workers it guaranteed cheap labour to the Afrikaner industrialists as well as to the capitalist farmers. This was the beginning of apartheid which provided a base for cheap labour:

> ...Apartheid, including separate development, can be best understood as the mechanism specific to South Africa in the period of secondary industrialisation, of maintaining a high rate of capitalist exploitation through a system which guarantees a cheap and controlled labour force, under circumstances in which the conditions of reproduction (the redistributive African economy in the reserves) of that labour force is rapidly disintegrating (Wolpe, 1972, p.433).

Desmond (1978) highlighted the myopia that afflicted even those who opposed the apartheid system. They did not see the role of capitalism in the origins of apartheid. The reason was that such people:

> ...accept the capitalist form of society as the normative one and the most obvious way in which South African society deviates from that norm is the racial nature of the forms of oppression; 'racism' is therefore presumed to provide the explanation for everything that is wrong with the system. It cannot be 'capitalism' because they start from the assumption that there is nothing wrong with 'capitalism', it can therefore only be 'racism'. That this does not in fact provide an explanation escapes their attention because they unquestioningly accept the capitalist analysis of the South African social system. But it is also the consequence of their

'idealist' understanding of the truth which assumes that people's behaviour is determined by their knowledge or beliefs. This understanding leads them to be primarily concerned about people's mental attitudes. Since 'race' is the cause of the problem and since behaviour is determined by attitude, the whole problem is one of racial attitudes and the solution is to persuade them to change these attitudes (Desmond, 1978, p.20).

If Desmond is critical of idealists, he is equally critical of Marxist interpretations of the apartheid system:

Radicals on the other hand, tend to dismiss all ideological factors and attempt to fit the "facts" into rather rigidly preconceived theoretical frameworks. Much of the debate centres around the conceptualisation of the problems and less attention is paid to new empirical evidence. Indeed many of the facts adduced by these authors are somewhat over-simplified (Desmond, 1978, p.25).

Desmond viewed South African capitalism as having two faces. There was the face of state capital which was under the control of the Nationalist Party and private capital controlled by Anglo-American industrialists, most of whom were members of the Progressive Party. In contrast, the face of private capitalism was not dependent on government intervention to maintain economic domination, and the growth of African political power was not a threat to them since they could have used other means to advance their interests. More important to private capitalists was the fact that a strong black middle class in urban areas would not only increase the market for consumer goods but would also act as a strong buffer between the rest of the working class, both black and white, and the capitalist class. This is why, Desmond asserts, from as early as the 1920s these industrialists started campaigning for African urbanisation and were opposed to forced removals. In contrast, state capital, mainly Afrikaner business, greatly expanded under the patronage of the Nationalist government. The position of the white working class was protected by purposive government intervention, not least the colour bar in employment which reserved certain jobs for white workers. The growth of the African political power would have inhibited the State from maintaining these interests hence the need to suppress all forms of African protests through extra-economic measures enshrined in the apartheid laws and regulations. The Nationalists encouraged the emergence of a black middle class, not in urban areas, but in the 'homelands'. Since this middle class would be composed of African employees in government service, it was hoped that it would support the status quo and act as a buffer between the rest of the black population and the white community. Desmond stressed that the resettlement policy was not:

> ...on the one hand, the work of demented racists, nor on the other, is it simply a result of the development or production in the dominant sectors of the economy. Rather it is a complex, comprehensive and effective way of exercising political control, arising from the present form of South African capitalism as a whole (Desmond, 1978, p.10).

Such a backdrop draws attention to the knowledge that the demise of apartheid, in itself, is not enough to bring about changes that would improve the health of the nation. The government has to tackle the fundamental causes of ill health and that is capitalism with its associated inequalities. In the health service inequalities date back to the arrival of white settlers when health services were developed to meet the needs of the ruling class.

References

De Beer, C. (1984), *The South African Disease: Apartheid Health and Health Services*, South African Research Services, South Africa.

De Kiewiet, C.W. (1942), *A History of South Africa: Social and Economic*, OUP, 1950.

Desmond, C. (1978), *Lunehill Revisited*, A Working Paper (later published by the University of Natal in 1978).

Wolpe, H. (1972), 'Capitalism and Cheap Labour Power in South Africa', *Economy and Society*, vol.1, No.3, pp.425-454.

2 The Development of Health Services in South Africa

De Beer makes the compelling assertion that historically health services in South Africa had no rational development. They emerged in the process of meeting the particular needs of the ruling class. Hospitals, for example, were established for sailors who worked for trading companies that came via the Cape of Good Hope. They were also built to accommodate and segregate people who were suffering from diseases such as leprosy, smallpox and other plagues which, it was feared, would infect the residential quarters of the rich and the powerful.

The first hospitals for black people were built in the nineteenth century by Sir George Grey - one in Pietermaritzburg in Natal, and the other in Kingwilliamstown in the Cape province. The motivation however, as the superintendent of Kingwilliamstown explained, was less to provide a needed health service than to ensure the allegiance of black people to the government of the day:

> Give me only one institution like this, give me talent and ability combined with kindness and mildness...let pure untainted charity have free play...let the heathen feel as free as in his own kraal...Such an institution will draw the savage from the remotest part of South Africa and attach himself forever to that Government which entered in spirit into his sickness and provided a remedy (De Beer, p.17).

Similarly, the development of a network of hospitals for mine-workers was a response to the prevalence of diseases such as silicosis and TB as well as industrial injuries among workers. Right up to the twentieth century the health of black people received very little attention. In 1920 the Government set up a Committee to 'Inquire into the Training of Natives in Medicine and Public Health'. Again here the concern, as the report from this Committee shows, was not the health of black people per se:

> It cannot be denied that at present there are hordes of Natives in many centres who have little chance of medical treatment and the untreated sick

6

become a menace to the community. Indeed, not just a menace but a double menace to South Africa. First, there is the immediate danger of the risk of infection and contagious diseases from areas where they may be said to be endemic. Second, there is the economic danger of the deterioration and eventual failure of the labour supply (De Beer, p.21).

The outset of the Second World War heralded further declines in the health situation for black people. In response to the war efforts the economy expanded rapidly with the national income increasing by 300 percent between 1933 and 1947. By 1939 the value of manufacturing had grown by 140 percent and by 1945 by another 140 percent. This expansion was accompanied by changes in the social structure with inherent political and social consequences. Between 1933 and 1939 the size of the black working class was doubled by the entrance of 400,000 people into the labour force. Most of the people moved into urban areas where there was already a shortage in housing. Acute overcrowding and low wages meant that for most black people life was a relentless struggle. These conditions facilitated and nurtured the development of black trade unions so that by 1945, 40 percent of all black workers in commerce and private industry were members of unions. The militant posture of the black labour force unsettled the government and it used its emergency war time powers to ban the black trade unions. The social dislocation of black employees with its attendant conflict emerging from rapid urbanisation persisted. The Smuts government did not know how to deal with this new situation and so it resorted to the creation of Commissions. One Commission under the chairmanship of Gluckman in 1942, looked at health issues. As De Beer points out, the health needs of black people had not resulted in a belated gesture of reparative altruism.

> The Gluckman Commission was appointed not simply because the government suffered pangs of conscience about the increasing number of sick people needing treatment. Rather, the level of disease was itself only one symptom of a society in crisis. Commercial and industrial interests and their political representatives in government attempted to contain this crisis through reform aimed at undermining the growing militancy of the urban proletariat. Improving health services formed part of this strategy (De Beer, p.23).

The Commission reported on the co-factors of scarce resources, the chaotic and uncoordinated health system, with an array of providers such as provincial, local and public health authorities, charities, including church-based ones, the mines and private doctors. The plight of black people was narrowly highlighted with the Commission stating '...native hospital needs go largely unsatisfied' e.g. a black hospital in the Johannesburg area, built to house 400 patients was used by 700 people. In South Africa there was one bed to every 304 white people and one to every 1,198 black people. In Cape Town the Commission found that there was one doctor to every 308 white people and one to every 22,000 black people. In Zululand and in the Northern Transvaal, the ratio was one doctor to every 30,000. It also found that 82 percent of the country's medical specialists were in big cities.

The Commission made a list of recommendations which included a free health service and the introduction of a National Health Tax to pay for the cost, a link between health centres and communities, health personnel, including doctors, to become state employees and the training of more health workers at every level. Above all, in respect of black people, the Commission pointed to the unequivocal social and economic factors in the causation of illness:

> ...unless there are vast improvements made in the nutrition, housing and health education of the people, the mere provision of more 'doctoring' will not lead to any real improvement in the public health. It would be unreasonable and unsound to expect the health service forever to make good the deficiencies of the socio-economic system. This achievement should be the goal of long term economic policy (De Beer, p.24).

In a sense, Gluckman was not merely ahead of Bevan, who created his National Health Service for Britain in 1948, but he also made explicit the link between health and social factors which waited until 1980 to be articulated in England (Black 1980). Gluckman had the sensitivity and insight to look beyond economic divisions and challenge racist and sexist attitudes which feed inequalities. He persuaded the Commission to recommend that:

> ...in the National Health System there shall be equal opportunity and equal pay for men and women performing work of the same nature...we wish to state emphatically that we are opposed to any selection which discriminates between one race and another (De Beer, p.26).

Even at a time when a woman's position was firmly believed to be in the home, Gluckman insisted that there should be no bar to the employment of married women. The recommendations of the Commission prove beyond reasonable doubt that the path taken by the many South African governments was not because they did not know what to do. The ideas on what to do to run the health service were far ahead of those in Europe. The government were not persuaded. So, as De Beer points out, the proposed National Health System was still-born. The government was not prepared to mobilise resources, the four provincial authorities did not want to let go of the control they held, the National Health Tax was never introduced, no attempt was made to make doctors State employees, and through their Medical Association doctors totally objected to free medical care available to all since this was going to interfere with their source of power, wealth and prestige.

In 1945 Gluckman became the Minister of Health and he made attempts to implement his recommendations. By 1948 he had managed to set up 40 health centres, and in 1949 the Institute of Family and Community Medicine was opened in Durban. However, these initiatives were given no financial or staff support so that by 1960 many of them had been closed-down and those which survived were handed over to provincial authorities who re-designated them as ordinary clinics. So, it came to pass, as De Beer points out that:

> the plan brought into the world with such hope, was finally buried. It would have been naive to believe that the Smuts Government could have implemented such a policy. Poverty, housing shortages and starvation are not accidental. They are inevitable consequences of a social order built on economic exploitation and racial oppression. A state based on such foundations would be denying its very nature if it were to produce a National Health System that treated its work force as people with human needs, rather than as economic units (De Beer, p.28).

The Smuts government was the 'enlightened' Progressive Party. This Party had some semblance of humane principles in its administration. When the Nationalist Party took power in 1948 the situation for black people in general, and in health in particular, deteriorated dramatically especially in rural areas. Under the apartheid system, thousands of people were moved into black settlements which had no facilities or employment. The pressure in the 'homelands', led to overspilling and the relocation of people into townships in urban areas. Here they established informal settlements of which Crossroads in Cape Town is the most well-known. Despite the vigorous application of the Prevention of Illegal Squatting

Amendment Act, the government could not resist the flow of people from rural to urban areas. In the 1980s the main movement was from white farms to homelands near cities. With increased pressure from political upheavals in the 1990s the movement was by-passing the homelands and people were creating informal settlements in urban townships even closer to cities, e.g. every month about 10,000 people from the Ciskei and the Transkei moved into Cape Town. It is estimated that half of the African population now live in these settlements. As a result the number of black people in Metropolitan areas increased from eight million in 1985 to eleven million in 1990 and this figure is predicted to rise to 23.6 million in 2010 (Critical Health, 1994). As a result of these relocations townships have become progressively overcrowded with associated health needs arising from the transition and the increased incidence of diseases.

The increase in population without matching resources created abject poverty in rural areas and many townships which accounted for high mortality rates among black people. In the 1970s, for example, infant mortality for white people was 15 per 1000 live births and the figure for black people was 100-110 per 1000 live births. Life expectancy for white people was 64.5 years for men and 72 years for women. For black people it was 51 for men and 59 for women. Even these are underestimations, argues Seedat (1984), because at least 50,000 deaths annually in rural areas are not registered. De Beer estimates that in the 1980s at least 15,000 to 30,000 black children died annually in South Africa from starvation or illnesses related to malnutrition. Many more died of gastro-enteritis and cholera as well as childhood diseases such as measles which pose less danger to children who are healthy. TB, a poverty-linked disease in this period, was rife. A survey undertaken in KwaZulu-Natal found that eight out of every thousand people had TB (De Beer, 1984). In the 1990s the situation nationally promised to become yet more explosive, with 90,000 new cases annually, and 3,000 people dying every year (Department of Health, 1996).

The inequalities underlying the causation of disease are also evident in the provision of health services in the 1990s. These inequalities are found between and within regions reflecting the patterns that existed under the apartheid system. As the following table shows, the distribution of registered general practitioners per 10,000 people in the nine provinces for 1992 reveals a bias towards the well to do areas (Jinabhai and Campbell, 1995).

Table 2.1 Distribution of GPs in the nine provinces

Provinces	Numbers of Registered GPs per 10,000 people
Western Cape	9.74
Northern Cape	2.98
Free State	3.43
Eastern Cape	5.54
KwaZulu-Natal	3.93
Eastern Transvaal	2.71
Northern Transvaal	1.41
Central Transvaal	6.94
Western Transvaal	4.07

Some of the names of the provinces have changed since these statistics were compiled.

Within the provinces there are further inequalities in the allocation of resources, e.g. the KwaZulu-Natal province has a population of 8 million people, a fifth of the country's population. The KwaZulu region of the province, which is mainly rural, has more people than the Natal region and yet it only receives four percent of the health budget allocation. The national average distribution of all doctors is nine for every 10,000 people. The Natal region which has cities – Durban, Petermaritzburg, Ladysmith, New Castle and many more - has 39, but when the KwaZulu region is included this figure drops to five. In 1992 there were 121 registered GPs in the KwaZulu region and in Natal there were 2,909. Further, there were three registered specialists in KwaZulu and in Natal there were 980. Even if account is taken of the fact that some doctors who have their registered addresses in Natal, work in KwaZulu, this does not bridge these stark inequalities. A further example of inequalities is evident in the distribution of the health budget (Health Policy Co-ordinating Unit, 1995).

Another example of inequalities noted by the Health Policy Co-ordinating Unit (1995), is in the geographical distribution of resources highlighted in the health budget of 1993-94.

Table 2.2 Geographical distribution of resources in the 1993-94 health budget

Province	Present Distribution (R000)	Equitable distribution (R000)	
Western Cape	2,109,396	872,956	-58.62
Northern Cape	248,164	210,502	-18.8
Orange Free State	992,657	971,226	-12.23
Eastern Cape	1,613,067	2,162,996	+34.09
KwaZulu-Natal	2,481,641	2,705,145	+9.01
Eastern Transvaal	372,246	903,772	+142.79
Northern Transvaal	620,410	1,772595	+177.65
PWV Area (Central Transvaal)	3,350,216	1,830,547	-45.36
North West	620,410	1,137,466	+83.34

Some of the names of the provinces have changed since these statistics were compiled.

Source: Health Policy Co-ordinating Unit (1995).

This was the inheritance of the ANC Government of National Unity when it replaced the apartheid regime in April 1994. There was overcrowding in townships where there were many square miles of shacks made out of plastic and cardboard. There was an estimated need for some three million houses. In 1995 running water was available to 98 percent Asian, 98 percent Coloureds, 100 percent Whites and 27 percent Africans, 15 percent of whom had to travel several miles to fetch that water from a communal tap. Only 30.5 percent of Africans had access to electricity as a source of energy in the household whereas almost all whites, Asians and Coloureds used electricity for cooking and lighting (Hansard 1996 pp. 3473-3474). In 1996 the National Sanitation Task Team (NSTT) estimated that 21 million South Africans had no access to adequate sanitation facilities. They still used buckets, open fields, unimproved pit toilets and poorly designed or operated waterborne sewerage system (National Sanitation Task Team 1996).

Poverty and lack of basic necessities remain major threats which combine to kill and disadvantage children. Already in 1993 Operation Hunger, an organisation involved in the feeding scheme, was sounding warning bells about the increase in the number of children who were affected by poverty:

In Natal, only 25 percent of these children are adequately nourished. Of the remaining 75 percent, more than 30 percent are in the red, the life endangered zone. The rest are stunted, underweight, part of the world wide ineducable majority who die by inches from the moment they are born. In the Northern Transvaal, we are seeing a huge number of malnourished children in rural hospital wards. One hospital had a 500 percent increase in malnutrition related illnesses. In the Orange Free State, the situation is far worse compared to that of 1992, with a 40 percent increase in clinically diagnosable malnutrition (Operation Hunger, 1993).

At the same time it was estimated that 17 million South Africans of all age groups were living in persistent and extreme poverty.

The government is not short of advice as to how it should deal with the problems of malnutrition. Operation Hunger made recommendations for urgent implementation including, interalia, free pre-natal care to all low income mothers, with food supplements if necessary, a pre-school nutrition programme for children from families below the poverty line, free compulsory education for all children from five to sixteen years, a re-introduction of State school feeding schemes, literacy and numeracy programmes for adult men and women, to improve their prospects of finding work, land for those whose lack of education gives them no alternative but to return to subsistence agriculture, housing projects geared towards South Africans with a family income of under R630 a month, a proper almoning system in hospitals and clinics, so that the poor can get free medical attention, reconsideration of the family planning structure and perhaps surprisingly, less 'capacity building', less 'co-ordinating', and more listening, in order to nurture and expand on the survival wisdom and hands on expertise of the people who were survivors.

References

Black Report (1980), *Inequalities in Health: Report of a Research Working Group*, Department of Health and Social Security.

Critical Health (1994), 'New Settlements, Growing Communities, the increasing need for health care', *Critical Health*, July Edition 46.

De Beer, C. (1984), *The South African Disease: Apartheid Health and Health Services*, South African Research Services.

Department of Health (1996), *The South African Tuberculosis Control Programme – Practical Guidelines.*

Hansard (1996), *Debates of the National Assembly*, 18 – 21 June.

Health Policy Co-ordinating Unit (1995), 'The 1994/5 Health Budget – Additional Resources Required', *Critical Health,* January, No.47.

Jinabhai, C. and Campbell, L. (1995), 'The need for Equitable Resource Distribution. The case for KwaZulu-Natal', *Critical Health*, January No.47.

National Sanitation Task Team (1996), *A White Paper on National Sanitation Policy.*

Operation Hunger (1993),Hunger and Death: Time to Act', *Critical Health*, December No.45.

Seedat, A. (1984), *Crippling A Nation: Health in Apartheid South Africa*, International Defence and AID Fund.

3 The Structure of the Present Health System

The vision for the present structure of the health service was laid down in 1994 as part of the Reconstruction and Development Programme (RDP) initiated by the African National Congress (ANC) in preparation for the functioning of the new government:

> The RDP is an integrated, coherent, socio-economic policy framework. It seeks to mobilise all our people and our country's resources toward the final eradication of apartheid and the building of a democratic, non-racial and non-sexist future (ANC 1994, p.1).

The establishment of the RDP was a necessary step in the transformation process. The racially determined inequalities outlined in chapters one and two were still in evidence in 1994. An important measure of this inequality was the nutritional status of children (see Table 3.1). The table presents the results of a survey of 97,790 primary school children with an average age of seven years, selected from 3,300 schools across the country (Child Health Unit, 1997).

Table 3.1 Primary school entrants with low anthropometric indices by racial groups

Racial groups	Sample size	% Stunted	% Wasted	% Underweight
Coloured	16,455	18.2	4.1	16.9
Black	65,511	14.6	2.4	8.7
Indian	2,559	4.1	5.2	6.2
White	2,024	1.4	0.8	1.1

Source: Department of National Health and Population Development, 1994.

These inequalities had their origins in the segregational policies of the apartheid regime which operated in every sector of society - education, employment, health, welfare, trade unionism, commerce and industry. To tackle such a shameful legacy six basic principles were adopted which, linked together, made up the political and economic philosophy underpinning the RDP:

- the RDP had to be an integrated and sustainable programme based not on piecemeal and unco-ordinated policies, but on strategies which harness and bring together resources in a coherent and purposeful effort that can be sustained in the future;
- it had to be a people-driven process to ensure the active involvement and empowerment of people irrespective of their economic status, race, gender or geographical location;
- peace and security for all is pre-requisite. This means the elimination of racist ideology and practices in the security forces, the police and the judiciary system, which in the past had supported the policies of the apartheid system. In turn, there is a need for personnel in all these areas to reflect the national gender and racial composition of society;
- nation building is required in which the iniquities which divided the country into 'first' and 'third' worlds are eliminated. The idea of developing certain sectors with the hope of a 'trickling down' effect for others was rejected since such an approach would fail to challenge the divisions laid down by the apartheid system;
- reconstruction was to be linked to development. Reconstruction, development, growth and redistribution had to form a unified programme. The unity was to be provided by an infrastructural programme which provides access to effective services such as sanitation, water, electricity, telecommunications, transport, education, health and training to equip people with a variety of skills. The aim of such integration was to:

    ...meet basic needs and open up previously suppressed economic human potential in urban and rural areas. In turn this will lead to an increased output in all sectors of the economy, and by modernising our infrastructure and human resource development, we will also enhance export capacity (ANC, 1994, p.6).

- The democratisation of South Africa aims at setting aside the minority control and privilege which had been the main obstacle to the development of an integrated programme. The democratisation process was central and indispensable to the whole RDP.

These interrelated principles formed:

> An integrated programme, based on the people, that provides peace and
> security for all and builds the nation, links construction and development
> and deepens democracy (ANC, 1996, p.7).

In order to operationalise these principles the RDP adopted programmes
which aimed at meeting basic needs, developing human resources, building
the economy and democratising the State and society.

Within this overarching enterprise health was given a high profile at
both micro and macro levels. There was a determination to improve health
services and a recognition that health problems have multiple and complex
causes, and that the promotion of good health requires a paced, interactive
and intersectoral approach. Within this approach, employment, housing,
clean water, sanitation and healthy ecological functioning were regarded as
having multi-level impacts on health.

Such theoretical and practical considerations fed and guided the process
of structuring the health service. It was in the context of this inclusive
vision that the framework for a single comprehensive system was
developed and it is to the structure of that system that we shall later return.

A Brief Review of the RDP Progress

The Health Systems Trust conducted a review of the South African Health
System in 1997. That review considered the perhaps premature progress of
the RDP. The reviewers noted that although the RDP was greeted with
much acclaim it was failing to deliver promises. Rather than seeing this as
a transitional problem that might be overcome, the authors took the view
that the failure was partly due to unrealistic goals which paralleled 'the
new government's wider inability to deliver on its election promises and
development programmes' (Van Rensburg *et al*, 1997). The Trust point to
such pervasive shortcomings in the implementation of the RDP as the lack
of integrated planning, inefficient delivery, lack of capacity, under-
spending, bureaucratic bottlenecks and protracted and inefficient
consultations. Even though values and principles which inform and guide
newly established policies and legislation were spawned by the RDP, the
programme was severely undermined by these shortfalls:

> Initially, the RDP received virtually universal political support. Within
> one year, however, this support had begun to erode, and within two years,

the separate ministry set up to implement the programme had been abolished, and the RDP thereby severely downgraded (Van Rensburg et al, p.24).

The RDP still has a role to play. Many housing projects are still funded through the programme. Nevertheless in the eyes of the people, it has lost the sparkle it had in its 1994 vision.

The Structure of the Health Service

One of the first priorities in the health sector was to draw together all different role players and services into a comprehensive health system. The government is on its way to achieving this objective but the system remains punctuated by divisions and turf-wars about who is providing what, when and how. One major division is between allopathy based on Western medicine and traditional healing based on African health knowledge. Under the apartheid regime the latter was officially banned from the national health plan and Western trained doctors, black or white, were in danger of being struck off the medical register if they included traditional healing in their practices. This ignored the fact that a large proportion of black South Africans were using the services of traditional healers. Thus legalisation had legitimised the antipathy towards African healing. The antipathy originated in the disrespectful attitudes and mind-set of influential practitioners imbued with Western concepts of disease and healing yet unaware of the extensive and long-standing role of African traditional healing. Deep divisions were fuelled by mutual suspicion and lack of trust and understanding:

> This is not in the interest of people who use all type of healers. The RDP must aim to improve communication and co-operation between different types of healers (ANC, 1994, pp.47-48).

To my knowledge this is the first time in the history of South Africa, since the arrival of foreign rule, that indigenous healing has been given legitimacy in a State document. That recognition, however, is not yet backed by the accompanying resources which would ensure that the service is available to all those who wish to use it in the same way that primary health care is used.

To a large extent the South African health service is very similar to the British National Health Service. This is not surprising since Britain ruled that country for a long time and many of those who make decisions about health and health-related issues were political refugees in England during the apartheid regime.

Health services are mainly provided by public and private sectors. The public sector is divided into (1) primary and (2) secondary health care. The former is provided through a network of clinics and health centres at community level and the latter in hospitals.

Primary Health Care (PHC)

In the Declaration of Alma Ata, PHC is defined as:

> ...essential health care based on practical, scientifically sound and socially acceptable methods and technology made universally accessible to individuals and their families in the community and country through their full participation and at a cost that the community and country can afford to maintain at every stage of their development in the spirit of self-reliance and self-determination (ANC, 1994, p.20).

The driving force in the transformation of the health service was to be the primary health care approach. Its emphasis is on the integration of preventative, promotive, curative and rehabilitation services in a climate which promotes community participation and empowerment in order to provide efficient and cost-effective health care. Unlike hospital services, where only certain categories are exempt from charges, primary health care is free to everyone. Primary health care services are provided in the community, in health centres and in fixed and mobile clinics which reach out to rural areas. For health purposes, each of the nine provinces is now divided into regions and each region has its own comprehensive primary health care team. At the time of the research, KwaZulu-Natal, for example had eight regions. In the course of this study I visited three clinics in Western Cape, three in KwaZulu-Natal and two in Gauteng provinces. I also had an opportunity to witness how mobile clinics work. In order to give some idea of how the system operates, I describe the structure and the functioning of one of the teams that I visited. Staff assured me that any differences between their operations and those of other primary health care teams are unlikely to be substantial.

The Structure of a Comprehensive Primary Health Care Team

The team works in the KwaZulu-Natal region. It is composed of six different but complementary sections under the directorship of a Chief Professional Nurse (CPN). Section 1 is the mobile clinic team. Section 2 is composed of three fixed clinics. Section 3 is the school team. Section 4, the sexuality/life skills team. Section 5 is the TB team and Section 6 is training. I will focus on Section 1 to which I was attached.

Section 1 is composed of five mobile teams, each with seven members of staff - a senior professional nurse (SPN), two professional nurses (PN), one enrolled nursing assistant (ENA), two enrolled nurses (EN) and one specialised auxiliary senior officer. (SASO). Each team is allocated four designated areas each with four meeting places where patients wait for the team. The teams go out from Monday to Thursday with Friday reserved for administrative work at the Centre. This means that each meeting place is visited once a month. The team met patients in the grounds of a local shop. When we arrived many patients were sitting on the veranda.

The meeting started with exchanges of warm greetings, a hymn and a prayer led by one of the patients. This was followed by a health education session, and the theme for the day was scabies and how parents can help minimise this problem in their children. It was obvious from the interaction that this was a familiar routine and not a special event to impress me. When the two professional nurses started their consultation in a makeshift tent and in the back of one of the vehicles, patients came out in the open to form a queue. This particular clinic was lucky in that the shopkeeper offered the use of one of his outer buildings which the team used for ante-natal checks, the weighing of babies and immunisation. Even though palpation was done with the woman sitting on a chair, it was better than doing it in the open air. On that day 154 people attended the clinic, 98 of whom received treatment - 32 children, 27 adolescents and 39 adults. According to staff it was a light day!

As patients were waiting to be seen I took the opportunity to talk to some individually about their health and what they thought would improve their health status. The answers pointed to micro and macro needs. Whilst people were appreciative of the service, they were concerned about its limited availability. They would have been happier if the team came more than once a month. Also, they wanted a building in which consultation could take place instead of standing for hours in the sun waiting to be seen. The day was blisteringly hot and on many occasions I sought the shade of the trees when I felt faint. There was agreement between the staff and patients that if it was raining the team would not come, but if rain starts in the middle of the consultation, then people get wet. At a macro level people wanted roads and transport. Some described how it took more than two hours to walk to the clinic. They wanted water, toilets, electricity and employment.

The work of the team encompasses curative, preventative and promotive tasks.

Curative This work includes the diagnosis and treatment of minor illnesses such as common colds, bronchitis, worm infestations, scabies, impetigo and the dressing of minor wounds.

Major illnesses are referred to doctors at established clinics or hospitals. Chronic illnesses such as hypertension, diabetes, asthma, epilepsy and TB are also managed by the team which prescribes repeat treatments that have been initiated by patients' doctors. But in the case of TB, a patient may have no need to see a doctor. If the team discerns symptoms that indicate the possibility that the patient may have TB, a sputum is taken and sent directly to the hospital. If it is positive the staff start treatment without referring the case to the doctor. The patient can be cured without having been seen by a doctor.

Preventative and Promotive Health Care This aspect of health care covers a wide range of activities performed by all team personnel. The work is focused on family planning, ante-natal care, child health, immunisation, health education and community projects.

The approach in this area is needs and client led. The activities inform and reinforce each other with the primary objective of improving the general health of people in the community. Health education focuses on the type of problems prevalent in a particular community and area. Where there is a lot of malnutrition, health education focuses on the use of locally grown food, how to grow and prepare it in ways that ensures their nutrition, particularly for the children. This information is then linked to family planning as the CPN explained:

> When we teach nutrition we also bear in mind that there is not enough food available to families. So we link this to family planning and explain to parents that if they limit the number of children through family planning then there will be less mouths to feed and the children will have less nutrition related illnesses. Bringing the two themes together enables parents to see the practical advantage of family planning.

Many community groups now have projects, and where there are none, the team encourages their development. Vegetable garden projects in particular are very useful in improving the nutrition which in turn promotes health. The staff who are there to give advice and support explain:

> Wherever we go we look to see if there are vegetable gardens. If there are none we encourage their development. We advise people what to plant and suggest that they make their own compost rather than buying chemical fertilisers. But we also have to check that people are not using the garden to plant maize and potatoes which they can plant in the bigger fields. We spend quite a lot of time. explaining the need to have vegetables in a diet. TB patients in particular must have fresh vegetables in their diet and to ensure that people do, South African National Tuberculosis (SANTA) gives all its TB patients funds to buy seeds. So all they need to do is to make the compost, till the ground and plant the appropriate vegetables.

There is a wide range of projects in which communities get involved in an effort to earn a living. But as the CPN pointed out, the people involved need the skills and the markets if what they produce will be the source of their livelihood. Where possible, team members operate as facilitators to this end:

> In one area we found that women had formed themselves into a sewing group producing different things which they were trying to sell to the community which has no money anyway. But we also noticed that the women were not very good in their sewing skills so we arranged for someone to train them. But then there was still the problem of the market. We then approached a hospital and suggested that they make a contract with the women to sew children's nightdresses, adult gowns, sheets, and bedspreads. The hospital stipulates the material and the pattern and the women provide them with a sample and if the hospital is happy with it, the women get the contract. This is working very well now with one hospital and we are now going to persuade other areas to follow suit.

The staff also encourage and support groups which have established themselves in catering. The staff explained that there are now many conferences and training sessions in which they are involved and there is no reason why these groups should not be given the opportunity to provide meals for the participants. But they stressed that such groups must be professional and efficient in their provision and they are willing to facilitate skills-improvement. Thus the staff are prepared to facilitate projects that enable communities and groups to earn a living in the knowledge that this will improve their health status.

Staff Training In order to provide this integrated service, staff require training. All staff have initial training which is supported by on-going, in-service training in their specialist fields. All staff must have a period of two weeks training in family planning. One professional nurse must take a TB course. All professional nurses take a health assessment and treatment course which helps them in the diagnosis and treatment of minor ailments and in assessing which patients need referring to a doctor.

Changes under the ANC Government

I asked the staff if there were any changes that had been initiated by the ANC Government and how those changes affected them and the people they served. The primary health care service pre-dated the new government but the number of mobile units had been increased from three to five to ensure that more people were reached. Even this increase is insufficient to serve the number of people who need them. Mobile clinics had always been free, people only paid when they attended at fixed clinics and the charge varied from area to area. In the fixed clinic for that area for example, people paid R3 per visit. Now all primary health care is free for everyone irrespective of location. Not surprisingly the team, just as their colleagues in the fixed clinics, spoke of the stress created by the shortage of staff. Each mobile team sees about 2,000 patients a month, a total of 10,000 from the five mobile units. Staff are also given targets which are used to measure the degree of their performance. Immunisation should account for 80 percent of all the people they see and family planning, 50 percent. To date the team has managed to achieve 60 percent and 32 percent respectively.

One problem hinges on the shortage of drugs. The free services had shifted a lot of people from consulting their private GPs to the clinics. The shortage is more acute in the supply of antibiotics. On many occasions patients arrive then leave without treatment. Transportation is a major concern. If the team was presented with a critically ill patient, there was no ambulance to transfer that patient immediately to a hospital.

A recent development introduced by the government is the establishment of Clinic Committees through which the community is given power in the administration and the running of the clinics. Apart from settling disputes between providers and patients, the committee employs ancillary staff such as security workers and cleaners. The government also gives money to the committees which then pay wages to workers on an hourly basis. The staff were not happy with this arrangement not least because it disadvantaged the ancillary workers. They received no benefits, had no days off or holidays and no sick pay since they were paid only for the hours they worked. There was a strong sense that this arrangement had less to do with the empowerment of communities than with saving money. It was conceded however that in the past, government funds had been eroded by the creation of ghost staff, by personnel officers who pocketed the salaries of non-existent workers:

> It was not unusual to find one person getting two or three salaries which were supposedly paid to staff that were never employed. So we do accept that the government must tighten the financial belt and procedures to stop such thefts. But this must not be at the expense of the most disadvantaged groups.

Some of the concerns expressed by this team were echoed in the other seven clinics I visited and are endorsed by a survey conducted by the Health Systems Trust in 1997. In their study of 160 clinics across the country, the average number of patients seen per nurse per month was 553. There was concern about the low availability of oxygen, a need to improve the supply of drugs, and a need for an ambulance service. On all indicators, the survey showed that rural areas faired worse than urban areas. For example, only 41 percent of rural clinics had an ambulance available within an hour of an emergency call compared to 74 percent in urban clinics and 59 percent in peri-urban ones (Health Systems Trust 1997).

It is important not to assume that the availability of ambulances is matched with access and service delivery. In the rural areas for example, the problem faced by many people is how to contact an ambulance service when there is no telephone service available in the area where they live. Even when there is a working telephone in the area (some local shops do have telephones) the clinic might not be able to receive calls. The survey found that in rural areas less than 50 percent of clinics had a telephone which was working consistently. To get to the clinic where they might be able to get an ambulance they have to walk long distances, sometimes lasting two to three hours.

In many areas transportation is hampered by the location of homes in areas which are inaccessible to vehicles. Immobile patients are carried or pushed in wheelbarrows to the road where the ambulance is waiting. However, urban and peri-urban areas have further problems vis à vis ambulances. Violence still has a strong presence in some areas, and the theft of cars at gunpoint has made ambulance drivers reluctant to go into such places. In addition, some places in the informal settlements do not have clearly identifiable addresses and ambulance drivers, particularly at night, have problems finding these places. However, the overriding problem common to the ambulance service as a whole, is the inadequacy of what is provided. Some GPs have described them as 'empty shells' with no life saving equipment. To improve the ambulance service all these factors have to be taken into account and addressed. The dependence of an efficient ambulance service on other developments, such as roads and telephone services, is also a very good example in support of intersectoral development for an efficient health system as outlined in the RDP. It is the responsibility of the Intersectoral Development Team to ensure that collaborative operation at every level, including the private sector, is a reality if good quality health care is to be realised.

The Secondary Sector

In the past hospitals were controlled by a variety of agencies. In 1994 the task of the government was to consolidate hospital services within a single framework. At present hospitals are either teaching or non-teaching and the broad operations of both are the responsibility of the Department of Health. However, the legacies of apartheid linger with the quality and the efficiency of hospitals largely determined by their users during the apartheid period. Hospitals that were designated for black people remain poor and under-resourced, and those which were reserved for white people have better standards. This is a general picture. One would also expect teaching hospitals to be better than non-teaching hospitals, not just in their curative capacity, but also in terms of patient experience. But this is not always the case. I visited eight wards in both types of hospital. I found some non-teaching hospitals to be very clean with a high standard of care for the patients, while others in the teaching category were wanting. In a ward that dealt with terminations, the situation was critical. The corridor outside the ward was full of women whose termination programmes had commenced. They were on drips and were carrying their own drip stands whilst waiting for other patients to vacate beds. There was no time for nurses to disinfect the beds before making them up for the in-coming patients. Some non-teaching hospitals have similar problems of demand outweighing resources. In one hospital where over 90 patients go through its casualty department, a nurse explained the routine:

> We see over 90 patients a day. The in-house doctor is an elderly man. He does not examine the patients. My duty is to ask patients why they have come to casualty. I then translate the information to the doctor who does not speak the language. He does not even look at the patient, he just writes down the treatment from what I tell him. But when a patient is seriously ill I ask her/him to get on the couch quickly and get undressed and then I drag the doctor to come and examine the patient. When a patient needs a drip, he lets the fluid drip into the patient's mouth instead of putting it in a vein. He is utterly hopeless, but there are no doctors around so they keep him on. In reality he should be struck off the register.

This shocking scenario speaks of senior level incompetence, lack of conscientiousness, absent commitment and ignorance with regard to the life-saving advantages and the appropriateness of intravenous hydration as opposed to oral hydration. But the bottom line is inadequate material and human resources.

People pay for hospital services. Outpatients pay R10. Manual workers pay R50 inpatient fee, provided they pay on the day they are discharged. If they don't pay on that day the amount doubles. All patients on Medical Schemes pay an inpatient fee of R403 a day. Fees for professional and business inpatients are determined by their salary but in general they tend to pay as much as those on Medical Aid Schemes. People who are exempt from hospital charges are children under six years old, pregnant and nursing mothers, elderly people, disabled people and some categories of chronically ill patients.

The Private Health Sector

In South Africa the private health sector is used by 20 percent - 25 percent of the total population and yet its estimated expenditure exceeds that of the public health sector. In 1995 the budget for the public sector was R 19.2 billion and that of the private sector was estimated at R22.7 billion (Health Systems Trust 1997). The private health sector has funders who pay for services, service providers who deliver health care and suppliers who provide equipment and drugs.

Funders

There are a number of different ways in which the private sector is funded. These include medical schemes, direct payment by individual patients to health practitioners, insurance companies, managed care organisations and medical savings schemes. Of these, medical schemes constitute the largest source of funding, accounting for two thirds of the total private sector funding and covering about 17 percent of the population. It is specifically for employed people since contribution to the scheme is from employers and employees. The amount paid is dependent on the individual's salary and the number of dependants.

Individuals also pay directly for private health services. These services include private hospital admissions, (about R465 a day), payment to doctors and for the drugs which they supply, (R80 for the initial consultation) and payment for over the counter medicines. In 1992/1993 funds from this source accounted for 23 percent of the total private health care financing (Health Systems Trust, 1997).

Providers

The majority of health professionals, with the exception of nurses, work in the private sector. The statistics taken from the Health System Trust Review, show that almost all pharmacists and a high proportion of dentists are in the private sector. The figures suggest that 58 percent of general practitioners are also in the private sector. Some of them also work in the public sector with the government paying the hourly rate.

Table 3.2   Health personnel practising in the private sector

Category	Total South Africa	Number in Private sector	Percentage in Private sector
General practitioners	17,438	10,067	57.7
Specialists	6, 342	3,657	57.7
Dentists	3, 748	3,330	88.8
Pharmacists	15, 794	14,841	94.0
Nurses	119,922	16,586	13.8

Source: Health Systems Trust.

Suppliers

The supply of drugs and equipment is dominated by local and international pharmaceutical firms. It is estimated that in 1996 the cost of the pharmaceutical industry was between 6 and 6.1 billion Rand. Drugs sold to the public sector accounted for 1.5 billion Rand and the private sector consumed 4.6 billion Rand (Health Systems Trust, 1997).

The over-concentration of human and material resources in the private sector has enormous implications for health care as many people are caught up between the poorly resourced public sector, at both primary and secondary care levels, and the prohibitive cost of the private sector. Two people's experiences, one in the Western Cape and the other in KwaZulu-Natal offer examples of what this means.

In the Cape Town area a man pushed his critically ill wife to a clinic in a wheelbarrow. The nurses who saw her decided that there was nothing they could do for her. She died outside the clinic, still lying in a wheelbarrow. The incident was the impetus for an inquiry into the working of the clinic system.

The second example concerns a woman who was admitted to hospital with cholera. She was put on a drip to replace lost fluid, but nobody attended to the fact that she was an insulin dependent diabetic. She went into a deep coma from which the hospital could not arouse her. When her sister, a trained nurse, visited her, she was told that there was nothing the hospital could do for her:

> I asked the doctor to write a transfer note so that we could take my sister to a private hospital. He refused and said there was no point because she was going to die within the hour. We decided to take her without his permission. We put her in the car and took her to a private hospital. Before they accepted her they wanted to know how we were going to pay for her accommodation and treatment. Had we not done that she would have died.

The second example is illuminating because the hospital was instrumental in creating the life-threatening situation. If the diabetes had been managed properly the patient would not have gone into a coma. What is troubling also is that the doctor did not seek to get the patient out of the coma, a task undertaken successfully in the private hospital. The health workers failed to focus on the whole person rather than the condition for which the patient was admitted. This was confirmed by a nurse's response when the woman's children who had arrived earlier than their aunt, pointed out that their mother was not responding to them:

I don't know what you are complaining about. Your mother came here with diarrhoea and we have given her something to stop it. What else do you want us to do? Just leave her to sleep, she must be tired.

If the staff had focused on her, her experience would have been very different. Her family need not have spent the vast amount of money on private health care. An unavoidable backdrop concerns the impacts of limited and impoverished services on employees. Staff morale in institutions with poor and inadequate resources has tangible implications in terms of patient care. Dedication and commitment are eroded when staff are over-stretched and do not have the means to perform their work.

Within the official structure of the health service, there is nothing between the public and the private sector. While not all public sector provision is as inadequate and as life threatening as the examples offered when emergency measures are called for, there is no means of access to the private sector, which has the resources, unless people have the money to pay for them. According to the South African Health Review, (1997) even those who are in the different medical schemes will soon be seeking care in the public sector because of escalating costs in the private sector.

One sector that has the potential to bridge the gap between public and private provision is the voluntary sector in the form of (Non-Governmental Organisations) NGOs.

Non-Government Organisations (NGOs)

There are 50,000 known NGOs operating in South Africa. These are developmental in nature (Health Systems Trust, 1997). During the apartheid period NGOs played a crucial role in supporting deprived communities at every level, including health. They came together and joined forces with other agencies in the struggle for liberation. In preparation for democratic rule, many NGOs worked closely with the potential government structure on policy formulation. The National Progressive Primary Health Care Network (NPPHCN) was heavily involved in the initiation of the Primary Health Care Approach. However, in the post-apartheid era some tensions have arisen between the government and the NGOs, despite the fact that there is still collaborative work especially at policy level.

The extent and the origins of that tension was communicated by a Director of Primary Health Care in the Western Cape who was to meet community groups soon after our interview. The interview hinged on (1) how far the government's health policies had been implemented and (2) the role of NGOs in that implementation in the area for which the Director had responsibility. Problems existed at both levels and they were financially based. In the previous two years, the Province had embarked on the building of new clinics as specified in the government's policy document. However, the parallel policy of equity in the distribution of the health budget resulted in Western Cape, which in the past had enjoyed an abundance of resources, making drastic cuts. All building programmes were stopped, leaving the province with only 20 new fixed clinics. Whatever finances were available were used to maintain what was already in existence.

Under the apartheid system, many of the NGOs received their funds from internal and external trusts. Under the ANC government many funders routed their contributions via the government. As a result many NGOs closed down. Even though the government wants to support them, it has not enough money to do this effectively. The Director said of NGOs:

> They are doing a fantastic job. They are there with the people for 24 hours. They have been doing this work for a very long time so they know what they are doing. The backbone in this area is done by people with minimum qualifications but who remain vital in this concept of comprehensive health care. And yet, we find difficulty in finding resources to support them. At the moment the best we can give them is moral support.

The Director was convinced that the success and the future of a comprehensive health care system lies in the government contracting with the NGOs. But there would be problems, some of which were already surfacing. Having worked independently in the past, some NGOs are not keen to be accountable to the government for their activities. Is it realistic therefore, the Director wondered, to give groups money if they are not prepared to show how those funds have been used and to what effect?

Some observers of the tension argue that the reluctance of NGOs to be firmly linked to government structures has little to do with not wanting to be accountable. Viewing the health service under the ANC Government they are concerned that it is already crippled by a culture of hierarchy, indecision, and lack of initiative, over-centralised, expensive and unresponsive to the needs of the majority (Grant, 1995). If NGOs were fully drawn into the state structure they would be disadvantaged by the same culture. Others argue that there are differences in the way groups perceive success in a project and that perceptions are based on the way development is conceived. Three main models influence that perception - growth centred, spend and service and people/community centred.

Growth Centred In this model the focus is on production, and success is measured in terms of quantitative growth. The co-option of local leaders is considered to the extent that they are prepared to operationalise the stated goals. There is little consideration of basic power relationships, a situation which can lead to the manipulation of the community through its own leadership.

Spend and Service Success in this model is measured in terms of the extent to which indicators of deprivation such as poverty, unemployment, homelessness, malnutrition and poor health are addressed. Although local participation is genuinely sought, it is not embedded in planning and decision making. Some material needs may be addressed, but there are no resources to build the long-term capacity of the local community to continue the work on a long-term basis.

People/Community Centred The emphasis in this approach is on process rather than the project. In the process of meeting basic needs, people are empowered with skills, knowledge and the capacity to act and engage effectively at the community level. Members of the Johannesburg Child Welfare Society suggest that State structures and welfare organisations in general, tend to adopt the first two models which stifle genuine community development through their maintenance of the status quo and social control. Instead of empowering people they create dependency and a sense of gratitude to the funders of the project. Their endeavours are doomed to be compromised as the link between development and education is ignored. Development, they state should be:

> ...a process of change that enables people to take charge of their destiny and realise their full potential. It requires building up in the people the confidence, skills, assets and freedom necessary to achieve this goal. True development is done by people, not to people (Johannesburg Child Welfare Society, 1993, p.85).

The Welfare Society offers what should be the hallmarks of a people-centred development project. It states that community participation must be evident at all stages of the project - planning, decision making and implementation - all according to the needs of the community. The ownership of the project by the community must be encouraged from the start and training in management skills must be a feature if development is to be a reality which enables people to be active participants, critical thinkers and creative problem solvers.

Thus agencies initiating projects must learn to let go in order to allow the community to develop the project in accordance with its needs. There is a perverse incentive for agencies to hold on because they want to show funders what they are doing. In turn, funders want to see results according to their own indicators of success which may be far removed from the impacts of projects.

What the Welfare Society calls 'the community worker's dilemma' is also the government's and the NGOs dilemma and one that must be resolved if services are to reach those who need them in the community. There is no doubt that development must be community centred in order to empower people but there has to be accountability to the funders, be they government or private trusts, and also to the beneficiaries of the project. Any organisation which provides money for a specific project and then does not want to know if that project has met its own objectives, is irresponsible in its administration of public funds. The issue is not solely about accountability but about objective setting. Once the goals have been set, there is an obligation for all concerned to see that objectives are met. There must be an understanding that projects are not static, i.e. they may prioritise, de-prioritise and add to objectives in response to the local context and emerging lessons.

If the potential of NGOs is to be realised in health services, then the government and NGOs must find a supportive working relationship in which the former does not control but is informed of the latter's activities and the extent to which set objectives are being met. Further, healthy communication is crucial in ensuring that funds are effectively used and that there is no duplication of services. Before that relationship is developed improved attentiveness has to be paid to mutual trust and improving understanding of mutual priorities.

Traditional Healing

Some observers would conclude that the inclusion of traditional healers in the RDP framework is a pragmatic rather than an enlightened vision about the role of African medicine in the treatment and prevention of illness.

My speculation finds confirmation in Gumede's observation in relation to the slogan 'Health for all by year 2000':

> It is a worthy cause but the responsibilities of this call are tremendous. The call implies the harnessing of vast resources in manpower, funds, skills etc. Technology is very costly to buy. It takes seven years and about R100,000 to produce one doctor, and about six years to train a professional nurse capable of meeting the needs of a primary health care facility solo in any rural area. The bulk of South Africans live in a Third World situation. If health for all be a reality by the year 2000, it is crucial and urgent that alternative health care systems other than the Western model be explored. Traditional healers are as old as Africa. China has had her 'foot doctors' for centuries. These are known existing resources (Gumede, 1990, p.iii).

The need to bring traditional healers into an integrated health system has been intensified by the HIV/AIDS epidemic. There are two aspects in this need. One relates to some of the methods traditional healers employ in the treatment of their patients, in particular ukuchaza (inoculation) with the use of razor blades. Typically, a healer will use the same blade with all members of the family without washing it. This has been identified by health workers as a mode through which transmission of the AIDS virus can occur. Most of the working links between the healers and the health workers have involved educating the former on offering health services without endangering lives. The other aspect concerns the search for a cure for AIDS. Some traditional healers claim to have found a cure. At a time of global investment in the search for a cure, the traditional healers are aware of the negative financial implications if their cure falls into the hands of unscrupulous researchers. The down side in this of course is that if they really do have a cure, nobody will know what it is and that means a great loss to African knowledge and human lives globally as the epidemic carries many to early graves.

Another possible explanation why the government is keen to include traditional healers in the scheme of things is that it is already faced with a 'fait accomplit' since, as Gumede points out, a large proportion of people use African medicine:

> The traditional healer, long spurned by Western medicine, and described with opprobrium as a 'witch doctor' and a purveyor of superstition and medical hazards, is constantly playing a larger role in today's medical care services, with or without licence to practise. Over 80 percent of black patients visit the traditional healer before going to the doctor and

the hospital. No records are available for those patients who are restored to good health by the traditional healer without visiting the hospital and/or the medical practitioner (Gumede, p.iii).

The importance of traditional healers is endorsed by the World Health Organisation (WHO), a body which still holds a lot of sway with governments of the world, health officials and professionals. From its own statistics, WHO affirms that two thirds of the world's population receive its health care from traditional systems of medicine, over a third of births in the world are delivered by traditional birth attendants, and in some rural areas, over 90 percent of births are delivered at home by traditional birth attendants. WHO expresses its approval when it states that:

> The healer and the patient belong to the same cultural group, viz, the same community and thus the prescription of the traditional healer is culturally meaningful and psychologically effective (Gumede, p.203).

A more positive view of the inclusion of traditional healing in the health plan is to suggest that the government is accepting the validity of culturally-based knowledge in health care and is recognising that Western based medicine has its roots in African medicine (Torkington, 1994). For the government to endorse Western medicine whilst ignoring African healing is like nurturing a baby whilst leaving the parent to die out in the cold, except that this particular parent refuses to die, and continues to nurture over 80 percent of its children who come seeking health care:

> Western medicine has official and government backing. It is dejure, but is there any basis for claiming any legitimacy on a de facto basis when 'traditional systems of medicine' remain the major source of health care for more than two thirds of the world's population? (Gumede, p.209).

Traditional healers have been fighting for recognition from the government for the past 50 years. Sazi Mhlongo, president of the Inyanga National Association, makes a distinction between genuine practitioners who want recognition for the vital role they have in the medical field and the 'sharks' who pose a danger to people's health:

> We have always been regarded as witchdoctors and as people without credibility. We have not been recognised for our contribution to the health field by the Department. For this reason there has been many

people who lost their jobs one day, and set themselves up as sangoma, inyanga or faith healer the following day (Sunday Tribune, 1997).

The reason why 'sharks' can operate is because there is no system to ensure accountability and it is for this reason that traditional healers want government backing in forming a Registration Council along the same lines as the Medical and Dental Council to ensure that those who practise are qualified practitioners.

The registration of traditional healers has the potential to discourage charlatans and to encourage training (Mhlongo, 1977). The request, valid though it may be, reminds one of what happened in Europe when registration was introduced. Many medicine women were killed as witches. Even now we remain inheritors of a medical system which exerts a lot of control on how we perceive and respond to our health needs. It is a system within which practitioners, tricksters or not, are generally protected by the cloak of clinical autonomy, legitimately conferred on all registered medical practitioners.

The theme of traditional healing will be re-visited when we look at how rural women in the Vulamehlo district approach this issue of power in the healing process. The following structure is presented by Gumede, a medical doctor, whose knowledge in this field comes from within his own cultural setting as a black person and also from studying the system of traditional healing in relation to Western medicine in which he is trained. The structure is given to enlighten all those people who still believe that all African traditional healers are witch doctors.

The Structure and Sectors of Traditional Healers

Destructive and evil	Abathakathi=wizards and witches
Diagnosticians or diviners	Izangoma, Izanusi (smellers), Abalozi (ventriloquists)
	Amandawu and Amandiki
Therapeuticians	Izingedla=Medicine men
	Izinyanga zamakhambi = Herbalists
Specialists	Izinganga zezulu = skyherds
	Izinyanga zemvula =Rainmakers
	Izinyanga zempi = military doctors
	Chief's special physician, Heart specialist, Kidney specialist, Chest specialist

It does not need extensive research to know that much of what was intended for post-apartheid South Africa has not materialised and critics have not been reticent about the reasons why the RDP has not delivered what it promised. This, however, must not eclipse the gains attained through the establishment of RDP. The Health Systems Trust points to one of these gains:

> ...many of the values and principles of the RDP became deeply enshrined in newly established policies and legislation. In particular, health and development policies of the post-apartheid era have been cast in the RDP mould (Health Systems Trust, 1997).

The suggestion here is that the intentions may not have been fully realised but the foundation has been laid and there is a hope that in time, what was intended will be fulfilled. Indeed, many call for patience, in the belief that change will not take place overnight. Others, however, argue that it is not just a question of time but the direction being taken. They point out that the government is not keen to re-distribute wealth for fear of upsetting the white population. Upsetting some people is inevitable. 'You can't comfort the afflicted without afflicting the comfortable' (Smith, 1990).

It seems appropriate to end this chapter with a quote which recognises the difficulties inherent in bringing about change:

> Drawing up a balance sheet on health and development in South Africa is no easy task. On the debit side, there is a lack of education, low economic growth, unemployment, lack of basic services and amenities, high poverty levels, inequalities in life-chances, social instability, crime and violence and the erosion of key social institutions and values. Superimposed on these are deep inequalities and disparities in most of the health and development indices, accompanied by severe deprivation. The imminent threat of HIV/AIDS is perhaps the most important single factor in the larger health and development game. On the credit side, significant progress has been made in a number of health and development areas including improving literacy rates, rising life-expectancy, falling infant mortality figures and greater immunisation coverage.
>
> As a result, South Africa's performance vis-à-vis Human Development Index is steadily improving. Most important in this balancing exercise, however, is the remarkable strides that are being made in the institutional reform of South African society. What is most significant in this respect, despite slow progress, sectional resistance and funding constraints, are the meaningful gains in freedom, democracy and equity, accompanied by the

systematic eradication of racism, discrimination and injustice. The hope remains that these gains will in time spill over to those areas of health and development which need improvement (Health Systems Trust, 1997, p.27).

References

African National Congress (1994), *The Reconstruction and Development Programme*, Manyano Publication.

African National Congress (1996), *A National Plan for South Africa*, African National Congress.

Cape Times, March (1998).

Child Health Unit (1997), *An Evaluation of South Africa's Primary School Nutrition Programme*, Health Systems Trust.

Gumede, M.V. (1990), *Traditional Healers: A Medical Doctor's Perspective*, Scotaville Publishers.

Health Systems Trust (1997), *South African Health Review*, Health Systems Trust.

Johannesburg Child Welfare Society (1993),'What is Development? The Community Workers Dilemma', *Critical Health*, December No.45.

Rex, G. (1995), 'Changing the Leopards Spots: The Quest to Improve South Africa's Health Service', *Critical Health*, January No.47.

Smith, A. (1990), *Journeying with God: Paradigims of Power and Powerlessness*, Sheed and Ward Limited.

Sunday Tribune, January 5 (1997).

Torkington, N.P.K. (1996), 'Black People and Science', in Torkington, N.P.K. (ed) *The Social Construction of Knowledge, A Case for Black Studies*, Hope Press.

Van Rensburg, D., Kruger, E. and Barron, P. (1997), 'Health and Development', *South African Health Review*, Health Systems Trust.

4 Children and Health

The survival of any society is insured to the extent that the society is able to nurture its children. In the previous chapters I have indicated how the black community under the Nationalist government, was systematically disadvantaged in this nurturing process. As a result, the health status of many black children was severely damaged. The effects of disadvantage are still evident today. Spotlights on malnutrition, learning difficulties, violence, with a specific emphasis on sexual abuse and political violence and mental health problems, consider but four manifestations of disadvantage.

The present government is aware that a healthy population is necessary for social and economic development. In order to have such a healthy population the government is determined to adopt development strategies which improve the quality of life of the population. For maximum effect these development strategies have to begin early in the life cycle. This chapter outlines the strategies adopted to eliminate the factors which threaten to cripple the nation at its very roots, its children.

Malnutrition

One of the socio-economic determinants of health is poverty. In South Africa poverty is racially and spatially distributed. Ninety five percent of the poor are Africans and seventy five percent of them live in rural areas. Many of the households in the rural areas are headed by young women, giving poverty a gender dimension. This is the legacy of the apartheid system, which was intensified by the forced removal of people from the land that they had occupied for generations. Some millions of people consisting primarily of the aged, the sick, widows, and women with dependent children, were dumped in areas with rudimentary layout for subsistence. The impact of those removals were revealed fully in the presentations to the Truth and Reconciliation Commission which I attended.

38

Children form the group most affected by poverty. Many children die of malnutrition and related diseases. Those who survive may be physically and psychologically damaged. The racial distribution of that poverty is reflected in the following table.

Table 4.1   Infant mortality rate per 1000 live births

Year	White	Coloured	Asian	Black	Total
1984	11.0	51.6	16.5	65.0	55.0
1985	9.2	41.7	15.4	64.0	53.5
1986	6.9	32.4	13.3	62.0	50.5
1987	12.3	51.9	19.9	60.0	51.7
1988	12.8	59.2	17.4	59.0	51.6
1989	8.8	39.4	12.7	57.0	47.7
1990	8.7	42.8	11.0	55.0	46.5
1991	8.6	38.6	11.0	54.0	45.3
1992	8.5	36.0	10.0	54.0	45.1
1993	8.4	33.0	9.0	53.0	44.1
1994	8.3	30.0	9.0	52.0	43.1

Source: Department of Health, 1994 - Health Trends in South Africa.

The statistics collected by Operation Hunger in 1993 show that malnutrition remains widespread in many parts of South Africa.

The health status of children, and the socio-economic factors determining it, has been the subject of many research journals and reports. The 1993 UNICEF Report on children and women in South Africa gave a situational analysis which covered children's mortality rates and trends, morbidity, malnutrition, HIV/AIDS, disability, education and development (Patel, 1993). In this section I consider what has been done to try and eliminate malnutrition.

To deal with poverty former governments in South Africa introduced a social security system under four categories: grants for elderly people, people with disability, child and family care and social relief. Originally these were introduced for white people but gradually they were extended to the whole population in amounts that adhered to the racial discriminatory practices. Within the field of child and family care, the main grant was the State Maintenance Grant available to means-tested women who, after applying through a magistrate's court, failed to get financial support from their partners or fathers of their children. It was also available to widowed or deserted women as well as women facing other conditions which imposed unacceptable levels of poverty (Lund Committee, 1996).

The Lund Committee states that although under the previous government all South Africans were eligible for the grant, African women were largely excluded from access. One of the reasons for this exclusion was that most of the independent homelands did not administer the grant system. As a result very small amounts of money were spent on the State Maintenance Grant. The figure for 1995 was R1.2 billion compared to R20 billion annually, if all women who were eligible for the grant were to get it. Within the Welfare Department this large amount of money projected in the above estimate raised concerns about the ability of the government to manage future payments of the State Maintenance Grant. It was this concern which led the Committee of the Minister of Welfare and the Provincial Members of the Executive Council (MINMEC) to establish the Lund Committee to investigate the problems around the Child and Family Support system.

Under the previous system a family received a maximum of R700 a month of which R430 was for the mother and R135 for each of the first two children. The Lund Committee suggested a replacement of this grant with a flat-rate child support benefit system.

The grant should be paid to the primary care-giver of a child according to a simple means test.

- it should be payable from birth for a limited number of years, with the number of years used as a cost containment mechanism;
- the level of the grant should be derived from the Household Subsistence Level for food and clothing for children;
- a condition for receiving the benefit should be the proper registration of the birth of the child, as well as the use of certain positive health related services;
- the money should be transferred on a quarterly basis into a bank or post office account from which it can then be drawn in any amount at any time by the primary care-giver;
- the benefit should be financed by the phasing out over a five year period of the existing parent allowance part of the State Maintenance Grant, and by not accepting new applicants for the child allowance part of the State Maintenance Grant (except for those who would qualify for the new benefit);
- welfare staff should attempt to divert women who will be affected by the phasing out of the Parent Allowance to training opportunities,

other departments should be asked to give such people special consideration when offering training and employment.

The government accepted the flat-rate and allocated R75 per child, an amount regarded as unrealistic by many welfare organisations which had lobbied for an increase in the amount. In response, the government increased the grant to R100 per child for any number of children under six years in a disadvantaged family. The new rate was implemented in January 1998 and will be phased in over a period of three years. It is estimated that the system will benefit 30 percent of the poorest children in the country. The Minister of Welfare and Population Development acknowledges that there are many more children who need the support but that financial constraints are a barrier. Following the advice of the Lund Committee the Minister announced that to prevent fraud by the people who administer the grants, money will be paid quarterly through banking facilities in post offices for rural women.

The increase has been welcomed by welfare organisations although they believe that the government has not gone far enough. The Johannesburg Child Welfare, for example, wants the grant to cover children of all ages:

> It is our hope that the government will in future allocate an appropriate portion of the national budget to social security for children of all ages because this would help us combat other problems, such as child labour and prostitution which result from destitution (Cape Times, 1997).

The South African National NGO Coalition which had suggested a flat-rate of R135 believe that the target of 30 percent would discriminate against a large number of people who are on low incomes:

> About 68 percent of children are living with caregivers who earn less than R250 a month. While we would appeal to the Minister to increase the target, it is close to impossible to find a means test, which is administratively viable, and cost-effective (Cape Times, 1997).

Despite these shortcomings the flat-rate system is one step in the right direction in dealing with malnutrition and its related diseases in children. The other initiative is the establishment of a Primary School Nutrition Programme (PNSP).

Following President Mandela's inaugural speech on 24 May 1994 in which he suggested a nutritional feeding scheme in every primary school which needed it, PSNP was implemented in September 1994. The programme has a number of related objectives. It is addressing problems of short-term hunger, micronutrient deficiencies, parasitic infestations and poor nutritional knowledge. A budget of R500 million was focused on needy schools in rural and peri-rural (informal settlement) areas. In its 1995 Annual Report the Department of Health states that approximately 5.5 million children in 15,800 schools received food supplements and more than 9,000 jobs and 8,000 project committees were created to operate the feeding at school level. Among the benefits which have accrued from the scheme, are improved school attendance, and income transference to parents as they have assistance with feeding the children (Department of Health, 1995). Despite controversies around corruption in the use of funds and the use of big companies in providing the meals instead of engaging local women, the feeding scheme has survived in many schools.

While there is no doubt that the scheme has a positive impact on the children who get the school meals the crucial period in the development of children, physically and mentally, is before the age of five. Since many children do not start school before they are five years old, a critical stage in intervention is lost.

The elimination of malnutrition and its related health problems in children can only be fully achieved with the establishment of long term supportive structures which begin at pre-natal stage. These should focus on the general elimination of poverty and the provision of adequate pre-natal care system. In the meantime there is a compelling need for intervention from birth to five years when the feeding scheme starts. The recently announced increase in the flat-rate child support benefit goes some way to addressing this need but since the target is 30 percent, many children will not escape malnutrition. This means that nutrition intervention programmes will remain an essential aspect in the social welfare provision for children under five.

I have come into contact with two schemes which work with children under five years, a crèche and a nutrition centre. I do not know how many other centres such as this exist in the country. What I describe below therefore relates to these two services. The Centre is called the Philani Nutrition Centre and is based in the townships on the outskirts of Cape Town.

The Philani Nutrition Centre

Philani is a community-based health and nutrition organisation which operates in a number of areas in Crossroads and Khayelisha. It operates independently and has a loose association with other NGOs which form part of the Progressive Primary Health Care Network. It works in partnership with other organisations such as civic and major health providers all of which are committed to providing a co-ordinated health care system. The original health centre was run on traditional lines with mothers coming in with their malnourished children who were suffering from a variety of illnesses. In 1980 the women health workers in Crossroads campaigned for a service that would realistically address the underlying causes of the illnesses - malnutrition. The first nutrition centre was opened in 1980 and since then several centres have been opened. Between them they serve about 500,000 people in the dense informal settlements covering about 3,200 hectares.

The Aims and Objectives of the Organisation

The organisation is committed to the protection of the rights of each child, to proper nutrition and health care and the right to grow and develop their full mental and physical potential. The Centre rehabilitates underweight children through a feeding scheme to counteract the crippling effects of short and long term malnutrition. The Director expressed her conviction that this is the most crucial stage in the development of the new nation:

> We have to intervene quite early in life before the damage to the children's health is done. Their physical, emotional and mental development is determined by the kind of nutrition they get when they are young.

It is this conviction which has led to the addition of two other projects, the Employment and Educare projects.

The Nutrition Project

Referrals for severely malnourished children come from hospitals in Cape Town, community health workers, clinics and day hospitals. In the centres children are assessed using a chart which is kept to monitor the progress of each child by a team including a nutrition worker, a nursing sister and a medical doctor. The mothers of the children come to the Centre and learn the principles of good nutrition hands-on by cooking breakfast and lunch for their children. Instead of expensive, high protein, Western style foods such as cheese, meat and fish, the ingredients used are those which are available at low cost and are familiar to the community. When the children have reached a certain level in their nutritional development, they do not come to the Centre anymore but health and nutrition workers visit their homes to monitor their progress. There is also a Health and Nutrition Education Programme within which health workers support mothers. They hold daily meetings in which they discuss health-related issues such as AIDS, TB, oral re-hydration and the benefits of breastfeeding.

The Employment Project

This project was initiated by women who came to the initial Centre. The children came for the whole day and women found themselves sitting around waiting to take their children home in the afternoon. Some women who had been involved in weaving schemes suggested that weaving should be introduced. The Centre now offers a training programme in weaving to all mothers who come with their children. The women make rag mats from waste fabrics bought from factories. The mats and wall hangings are sold in many craft markets in Cape Town. Others are sold to tourists who visit the Centre. The money goes directly to the woman who has made the artefact and a small amount is taken for buying the raw material. In this way, the project provides much needed income to impoverished families, which enables them to continue the nutrition programme at home. The aim 'is to run the Centre as an economically independent venture' with mothers and the Philani staff. Central in all this is the commitment 'to work for the empowerment of women by providing training opportunities leading to greater self reliance and confidence'. Not only are women learning weaving and selling skills but they have the opportunity to be together in solidarity and in support of each other.

The Educare Programme

This programme is geared to the stimulation of children's development. The focus is on their physical, social, emotional and intellectual development. They are also stimulated to develop their cognitive and language skills. The Educare workers who run the project are drawn from mothers attending the Centre with their children. They get their training from an established pre-school agency, the Early Learning Resource Unit. The qualification women get from this training enables them to run crèches and to foster pre-school education.

Most of the staff in the centres are drawn from the surrounding communities, 'a factor', stated the Director, 'which roots the centres in the local context and strengthens community links'. Women who came originally with their children have now been trained as Educare workers, weaving instructors, sellers, administrators and health and nutrition workers. Sixty percent of all workers in the centres had their first contact with the organisation as mothers of children who came for the rehabilitation programme.

The Director was very keen to develop more facilities for women. She was planning a women's health group:

> Women are very disadvantaged in all aspects of their lives. In the Centre we are going to explore every possibility to improve their lives. We have had a literacy project here, but I think the people running it have had some financial problems, so it has now stopped. But we intend to pursue this again in order to give women an educational chance.

Reflections

I found this an exciting organisation which was starting at the crucial stage in child development. It is acknowledged that not only do millions of black children in South Africa die before they are five years old because of malnutrition and related diseases, but even of those who survive, many are not fully developed physically and intellectually because of the starvation they experience in their early development. The future of South Africa and of black South Africa in particular lies in the capacity of the country to nurture its children and prepare them for their roles in its development. The Philani Centre project was not introducing expensive and sometimes unhealthy foods based on Western diets but on traditional foods which could be produced by people in their fields. They needed land to produce it and the distribution of land awaits government impetus.

The project had centres located within a 20-kilometre radius of each other. Each centre had contact with between 500 and 1,200 malnourished children and their families. The programme had been successful in holding back the onslaught of malnutrition on a large number of children who had used its services. However, making their achievements more widespread was not regarded as straightforward by some:

> Programmes work best when they involve mothers in education, when the nutrition intervention is linked to other local initiatives, and when there is a close feedback loop between a change in the mother's behaviour,

change in the nutritional status of the child and the response of the programme.   A programme such as Philani in Cape Town links its success on the nutrition front with the development of income-generating opportunities for mothers and other women.   Such projects, however, tend to be the outcome of a particular combination of circumstances at a local level at one time, such as the degree of community organisation, leadership, the presence or absence of other health services, etc (Lund, 1996, p36).

Whilst in general I accept the reservations of the Committee I do not think all the ingredients must be present at the outset.   Factors may emerge as a consequence or a response to developments within the project, i.e. in Philani case, the employment project which gave women income-generating opportunities was initiated by mothers whose children accessed the rehabilitation programme.   With regard to a favourable combination of circumstances, does this mean that a service like a nutrition centre cannot be replicated where it is needed because circumstances are unfavourable? Is it not possible to promote favourable circumstances in areas where there is a need to develop a similar service?   Recognition of the merits of community development and leadership skills provides important clues. Listening to people, responding to their expressed needs, encouraging the creation of factors which will ensure the success of any endeavour are as crucial as financial resources.   As the editor of Recovery observed, 'give people resources and they will do what needs to be done to meet their needs'.

Children with Learning Disabilities

It is acknowledged that the intellectual development of a child is dependent on the nutrients available to the mother before and during pregnancy as well as to the baby after birth.   We also know that in South Africa capitalism and apartheid have combined to deny many black children these nutrients at every stage of their development.   Many have died as a result of starvation and those who survive, as Operation Hunger states, are physically and mentally damaged.

Some evidence which links intellectual development and nutrition and therefore supports the above statement, comes from special schools which have children who they describe as 'slow learners'.   The children start in main stream education where they fail until they are sent to a special school where they join severely disabled children. The head teacher of a special school described the scenario:

> These children know that they do not belong here. When they are taken home after school they hide on the floor of the bus because they do not want people to know that they go to a special school. They will not get out of the bus if main stream school children are around.

The school I visited is the biggest in KwaZulu-Natal with 260 pupils. The Centre does assessments once children have been admitted. Children who turn out to be slow learners are given quality time and as their learning skills improve, they are given a chance to do mainstream examinations and if they progress well, get a chance to apply to main stream schools.

Before 1984 there were hardly any facilities for children with learning disabilities. Even now there are not many. The one I visited takes children from all over the province so it has 31 boarding pupils. There is a long waiting list and some children are not accepted because the age criterion for admission is 14 years.

Classes are determined by the learning capacity of the children. There are classes for the 'educable' who are taught mainstream subjects and other classes for the 'trainable'. Here they are taught basic skills such as eating, toileting, dental care and dressing, social skills, physical fitness, communication, co-ordination - catching a ball, dancing - and pre-vocational skills. There were also craft classes where children were taught woodwork, painting, and needlework.

When children reach school leaving age, many move into a workshop which is on the same premises as the school. Here they are streamed according to their ability and are paid accordingly. They make dog kennels, toilet units, benches, small tables, cupboards and also repair furniture. The firms that bring this work to the workshop pay the going rate to the Centre and the workers are paid by the Centre according to their production. Wages vary between R5-R33 a month in addition to the grant they receive from the government. No workers were employed at the firms' premises.

The staff in the school and the workshop are very committed to the welfare of the people they support. However, their contact ends when the children and the workers go home. They cannot address the fact or extent of the sexual abuse visited on their pupils and workshop employees.

Many of the children who come from children's homes have been sexually abused. Even those who live in their own homes are not safe. The bus picks them up in the morning and brings them back at 12.30 in the afternoon when parents are still at work. Some of them, left alone in the house, are raped by uncles, neighbours and family friends who are supposedly looking after them.

The staff estimated that at least ten percent of their pupils are sexually abused, some on a daily basis. Not only is this indicated by a change in the behaviour of the child, but the children say in detail exactly what has been done to them, and by whom.

This is not a new phenomenon. Since 1984 parents have been involved in arranging terminations for their children. Some of the parents themselves have learning disabilities, but even those who do not, experience helplessness in ensuring the safety of their children because of the way the criminal justice system deals with offenders. Even when there is a medical confirmation that the child has been raped, the court can and does throw out the case because children with learning disabilities may not be equal to describing what has happened to them. The perpetrators continue raping the children. Whilst the majority of raped children are girls, staff reported fewer incidences of boys being raped by women.

The staff are in anguish about what is happening to the children. They point to lack of resources to ensure the safety of the children whilst parents are out at work. The best they can do is to warn parents not to unquestioningly trust their friends and relatives.

Sexual abuse is not the only health hazard faced by children with learning disabilities. Many come from poor homes in which they have been malnourished and as a result have suffered from poverty related diseases. What is even more depressing is that many of the children face barriers within their own homes and communities because they are seen as 'different' and their human rights are not as legitimate as that of 'normal people'. Their health needs are hidden in the all embracing identity which focuses on learning disability rather than the whole person. Many of the children remain unlinked to their peers and sometimes their families. They have little access to health and have no voice advocating for their human rights.

Most black children in South Africa are disadvantaged in a number of ways by the legacies of apartheid. But children with learning disabilities are doubly disadvantaged and are likely to remain so unless there is a change in societal and communal attitude which will be measured by the quality of resources and opportunities made available to them.

Children and Violence

Statistics from the first national study of crimes against children conducted by the Human Science Research Council (HSRC) from July 1994 to June 1995 (Desmond, 1997) set the scene for this section.

Nature of crime

- 62% of the children were victims of crimes of a sexual nature;
- 14% of common assault;
- 11.1% of serious assault;
- 3% of offences under the Child Care Act;
- 2.5% of kidnapping;
- 2.3% of abduction;
- 0.6% of attempted murder;
- 0.3% of murder.

Relationship between offender and victim

- 83.5% of the perpetrators were known to the victim;
- 35.3% of the crimes were committed in the child's own home;
- 23.7% were committed in the offender's home.

Gender

- 75.4% of the victims were female;
- 88.9% of the offenders were male.

Race of the victims

- 44.3% were Black;
- 35.1% were Brown even though they make up only 2.4% of the child population;
- 19.26% were White;
- 1.2% were Indian.

Employment and Educational Status of the offenders

- 39.9% were unemployed;

- 17.9% were employed as labourers;
- 3.5% were high-income persons, such as professionals, mangers or executives;
- 4.9% had a post-school qualification.

The way the judiciary system dealt with offenders

- 62.9% had previous record;
- 63.2% were traced but were not tried for offence they committed;
- 7.4% received a prison sentence.

Counselling Services for victims

- 44.4% received no help;
- 41.8% were assisted by a social worker.

Future trends suggest that crimes against children will increase by 29 percent a year. If this trend continues, by the year 2000 the Child Protection Units will have to deal with 1,478,110 cases of child abuse.

Shocking and unsettling as these figures are, they are incomplete. Even within the criminal category, there is a huge discrepancy between cases that get into the records of the Child Protection Units and the numbers of children who are subjected to violent crimes. Many of those who are sexually abused do not see perpetrators reported, even when known by members of the family. Others are only known to the child and the perpetrator who creates enough fear to stop the child telling anyone. Discrepancies are also created by applying a narrow definition of violence.

Crime is not the only source of violence affecting children. The major source in the violation of children's lives in South Africa is economic. Most of the children thus violated are black. When children die because of poverty, when they are stunted, underweight and as a result they are damaged physically and mentally, that is violence.

Then there is environmental violence. When children lack good accommodation because of insufficient housing, when they have no recreation facilities, when they have poor schooling facilities, that is violence.

When children do not receive loving attention from their parents and society, when they are humiliated by the administration of corporal punishment both at home and school, that is violence. All of these fall under the violation of human rights and they are forms of violence insofar as they assault children's development potential. It is only when all these dimensions are layered onto the above figures that we can begin to understand the violence experienced by millions of children in South Africa. In this chapter the focus is on sexual and physical abuse in order to put into context the work of a centre I visited which uniquely supports children who have been abused.

Theoretical Perspectives on Violence

Many social scientists who have analysed the increase in violence experienced by children in South Africa point to an interrelationship between the public and the private spheres within which children live. For Campbell (1996) that relationship is mediated by a gender dimension which may explain why 75 percent of the victims are female and 89 percent of the offenders are male. Drawing from her interviews with older and younger men who were working class residents in a township in the Durban area, Campbell, argues that the wider social economic and political structure is heavily implicated in the creation of violence evident in the black community. Historically black men in the public domain were disempowered by capitalism and apartheid, leaving the family as the only arena within which men could exercise their patriarchal authority. But the shifts that have taken place in the last 15 years have created a climate within which the family is no longer an automatically available arena for the assertion of male power.

From the older men's point of view the factors responsible for these shifts include the erosion of intergenerational respect as younger people refuse to accept their authority since they can no longer fulfil the important role of breadwinner as a result of unemployment; the growing power of the youth in the political arena and the younger people's lack of commitment to traditional ways of treating adults which leads to bad behaviour. This loss of patriarchal power is seen to contribute to the increase of violence in older men. The younger men, on the other hand, argue that the problems of intergenerational respect have arisen because the demands of modern life in a township have made their parents incompetent social guides - they lack education and therefore have less status; they lack sophistication because of their rural origin; they lack political consciousness and they accept their humble work status. Young people, states Campbell:

...drew a sharp contrast between their parents' passive acceptance of racial discrimination and economic disadvantage, ...and their own active resistance to these phenomena... (Campbell, p.207).

Arising from this contrast young people have had higher expectations in their life chances which have been frustrated by unemployment and the slowness in political change. But unlike their fathers who found a niche in a family setting, young men cannot be inserted into a family life as husbands because unemployment means that they cannot afford to pay the lobola (bride wealth). The result of all this, is a crisis in masculinity:

> Violence in both the public and political spheres can be linked to a more general crisis of masculinity. Apartheid and capitalism have limited the power of working class men. Historically they have sometimes sought to compensate for this lack of power in the wider society within the context of the family, where they were able to draw on the notion of tradition to justify their power over both women and younger men. A number of factors have undermined male power within the family. Violence is suggested to be one way in which men attempt to reassert their masculinity in the face of numerous undermining factors (Campbell, p.213).

Ramphele picks up the same theme of the relationship between the wider structure and family dynamics when she analyses the violence faced by young black people in New Crossroads, an informal settlement in Cape Town:

> Young black people face the problems they do largely because society has failed them. Their families' capacity for nurturing has been eroded by the complex social forces which have conspired against them (Ramphele, 1996, p.57).

Henderson's contribution on the same theme is drawn from a three year research study from 1992 to 1994 on corporal punishment within families and in schools. In her interaction with children from 16 households she came to the conclusion that although the severe beatings that children endured were a standard form of admonishing children, they were also an:

> attempt to assert a particular organisation of power relations, with the beaten person forced into a position of deferential submission in relation to the beater or conversely to resist this (Henderson, 1996, p.79).

Although these power relations and the severe beatings that maintain them exist within families, we need to be aware that they are shaped in the wider sphere through daily practices within societal structures and that of individuals:

> ...the frequency, and in many cases, the severity of corporal punishment cannot be viewed uncritically, taking place as it does in a field of contested power relations. In transforming the lives of all South Africans and particularly those of children, we need to reflect on our culpability in shaping the realities in which we live by facing the outcome of our daily practices. It is through these daily practices that our agency is expressed, and where we shape our response to inheritance and global influences (Henderson, p.83).

Although the above scientists are specifically concerned with the situation in South Africa, their analysis falls within a general broader framework which puts at the centre of all forms of violence, power at both structural and personal levels. Waldby *et al* are proponents of this power theory. They assert that structural power is granted to individuals or groups of individuals by society on the basis of criteria such as age, gender, race, status and many others. In these socially accepted divisions, society legitimises the exercise of power over the powerless:

> This construct is a cornerstone of patriarchal hegemony and without it, aggression against and exploitation of people who have little or no institutionalised power (children, females, Black people, working class people, the disabled etc.) could not be maintained (Waldby et al, 1989, p.102).

The authors link this hierarchical power to personal power which in itself is positive in that it enables individuals to have control over their own lives and gives them inner strength to achieve their goals in life. It is a source of strong motivation to survive. However, in some people who have no self-worth this power becomes negative as it is rooted in fear and anger. Such individuals are prone to use this negative power to harm themselves or others. It is the combination of these two levels of power, argue the authors, which explain, the patterns of violence in any given society.

The link between structural power and violence is highlighted in the work of Straus, Gelles and Steinmetz looking at intra-familial violence in relation to child abuse in the United States of America (Straus, *et al,* 1980).

Corby summarises their explanation of the high rates of child abuse they found in their study:

> ...they argued that violence is a socially sanctioned, general form of maintaining order and that it is approved of as a form of child control by most people in American society. It can be argued from this perspective that a society that approves of the corporal punishment of children in schools and endorses the old adage 'spare the rod and spoil the child' sets the scene for a variety of unwanted forms of violence, of which physical child abuse is one. Thus, child abuse is seen to be on the same spectrum as socially approved forms of violence rather than as a separate pathological phenomenon (Corby, 1994, p.99).

Henderson endorses this and implores South African society to reflect on the acceptance of power relationships which legitimise child abuse because only then will there be a real transformation in the lives of all South Africans.

Whilst these explanations are useful I am mindful of generalisations. These neither tell us why some people under similar circumstances do not exhibit the same kind of behaviour nor why some do.

Child Sexual Abuse

In South Africa there has been an increasing concern about the rising incidence in child abuse, especially sexual abuse. In 1994 the Human Science Research Council reported that in 1993 there were 3,698 cases of child rape and in 1994 that figure had risen to 11,167. The statistics reveal that in 1993 sexual abuse accounted for 62 percent of all crimes against children and in 83.5 percent of cases the child knew the perpetrator (Desmond, 1997).

In 1995 clinics in Soweto, a black township on the outskirts of Johannesburg, were dealing with more than 100 raped children below the age of 10 a day. One district surgeon was handling more than 120 cases of abused children every month (Sowetan, 1995). Staff who attended to abused children in clinics reported that many of the children who had been raped exhibited high levels of psychological problems. In addition many were left with physical problems such as rupture of internal reproductive organs which may lead to infertility in adult life; they get infected with sexually transmitted diseases, not least HIV and AIDS, they get bone infections which sometimes produce paralysis from the waist down and they may also develop the loosening of pelvic muscles which may cause urinary disorders (Sowetan, 1995).

It will be recalled that South Africa provides a backdrop in which unemployed and ill-educated men feel frustrated and socially impotent. This does not account for the prevalence of child sexual abuse. Factors such as overcrowding, homelessness and hopelessness which exist mainly in squatter camps are strongly associated with degrading conduct which includes child sexual abuse (Desmond 1999, private communication).

Another factor to which many have pointed is the void created by the demise of the apartheid regime. During the Nationalist rule the struggle for black liberation had a positive psychological effect on people. Although there was still poverty people felt there was a purpose in life, something to live to fight for. Even those who were not fully drawn into this way of thinking, and were inclined to remain in the web of criminal activity, there were community structures such as street committees, people's courts and other civic groups that controlled crime in the townships. The dismantling of the apartheid regime, without a corresponding positive change in the lives of many people, has not only created a void, but has also dismantled some of the structures which kept crime under control. As a result, those who are left feeling hopeless, degraded and without purpose, have turned to crime and children and women are the most vulnerable.

There is a further angle to consider, informed by the analysis of the 'Battered Baby Syndrome' rediscovered in the USA by Kempe and associates (1962). They revealed that the phenomenon had existed for a long time but had remained hidden. I wonder how transferable their thesis is to rural communities. Having been brought up in a rural community where there was no privacy in living and sleeping arrangements, I find it difficult to see how child sexual abuse could have thrived undetected, not only by members of the immediate family, but neighbours as well, who walk in any house unannounced. Whilst I accept that abusers seek to avoid discovery, I wonder about the extent of sexual abuse in rural communities.

Some may argue that in South Africa child sexual abuse pre-dates the transition to democracy and the political system is responsible for hiding the phenomenon, i.e. that during the apartheid regime crime on black people, including child sexual abuse, was not given priority by a police force whose resources were devoted to political oppression.

Another reason for the apparent absence of the phenomenon in the past is the stigma it carried in the community which prevented people, including mothers, from talking about it. But now, Magidela points out, democracy in the new South Africa has given birth to freedom of speech, has empowered women and has given them confidence to speak out about what is happening to them and their children. In her report on child sexual abuse she quotes an angry mother whose child had been sexually abused:

> It is a blow to the heart - the man you love, your child, you want to spend your life with both of them as a family. It is more than death itself, because death passes. Sexual abuse of your child lives with you, it is like carrying a heavy stone on your back and walking miles. You look at the child and wonder what kind of a mother she will be. Every mistake she does you associate with the effects of this abuse, you live with the blame, it destroys your life completely. There is this thing knocking in your brains, your life is totally destroyed, you are just a walking corpse (Magidela, 1996, p.22).

The quotation confirms Magidela's views and belief that as more women become confident to report the sexual abuse of their children this will be reflected in the statistical data. McKerrow, a paediatrician specialist, offers another reason why there will be a rise in reporting sexual abuse that is linked to the HIV/AIDS epidemic. The virus in South Africa has created numerous fears, myths and legends - some rational and others with no scientific base. McKerrow described three myth-based theories that link child sexual abuse to HIV/AIDS - prevention, cleansing and retribution.

The 'prevention' theory relates to the general fear that people have about contracting HIV. To avoid the virus, a man will seek to have sex with an uninfected person, preferably someone who is not yet sexually active. People who fit in this category are children between four and ten years old. Thus children in this age group are targeted for safe sex.

The 'cleansing' theory is about getting rid of the HIV virus or AIDS. There is a belief that if an infected man has sexual intercourse with a virgin, he will pass the virus to the woman and thus leave himself free of the infection. As a matron in one of the clinics dealing with child sexual abuse stated:

> There is a belief that having sex with children from 9 months to ten years old, who still have a hymen, will stop them from dying of AIDS. But this is not true (Sowetan, 1995).

The final theory is about retribution which McKerrow believes holds sway in peri-urban areas:

> This theory reflects a belief, very prevalent in peri-urban settings, whereby individuals who know, or believe themselves to be infected deliberately try to spread the infection to all sectors of society. Whether this is a response born of anger or a desire for revenge, or a reflection of unity amongst marginalised youth, where both triumphs and setbacks must be shared, is uncertain (McKerrow, 1996, p.5).

The deliberate spreading of the virus is a phenomenon confirmed by health professionals interviewed in this research. It is a real problem to which no encouraging solutions have been found.

What we have is a collection of theories to which many more can be added. The women in Magidela's study pointed to loosening cultural ties and the abandonment of customs, the migratory labour system which destroyed the extended family and substituted it with smaller family units; separation of spouses, leading to single parenting and lack of education, in particular religious education which has been weakened within the family and society at large:

> Any human behaviour is structured according to the laws of God, but most people, especially men, have turned away from the way God structured nature. Even the government is ruling according to the laws of man. This is where everything went wrong. People are not being governed on the basis of Christianity, that is why they do not think deeper or use their reasoning in conducting their behaviour (Magidela, p.23).

I do not think any one theory can give us the answer. The explanatory power lies in their collectiveness and interconnectedness which allow emphasis to be put on some in different circumstances. Whatever the causes of child sexual abuse, its effect on children, as I learnt when I visited the Luthando Centre, is horrendous.

Luthando Centre (a place of love)

In Orange Farm, a community faced with immense poverty and overcrowding in shacks, where one small room is made into two using curtain dividers, the problem of child sexual abuse is acute. The situation is aggravated by the slowness with which the police and social workers deal with cases of rape. It is this lack of quick response which led the women in Orange Farm to establish Luthando Centre.

The Centre served as an interim trauma clinic which took in sexually abused children away from the scene of abuse whilst waiting for the police to deal with the crime and social workers to find a place of safety. The whole process was started by one woman, Mrs Mooi, a pensioner, who took raped children into her shack home. Later the women received some funding from Royal Netherlands to build a hall where the children could stay. When I visited the Centre there was no one in residence because Mrs Mooi kept the only child who needed accommodation at the time at her house. The Centre had 12 beds and nothing else. The floor and the walls were concrete and the place was ice cold. The cooker and the fridge, donated by the Netherlands Trust, were kept in the Mooi house where food for the children was cooked. One of the problems was lack of money. Mrs Mooi explained why:

> At one stage I had seven children here for the whole week. I had to use my pension money to feed them. My husband is a pensioner too, so we really do not have money to spare. Under the new system each child should have a voucher which entitles her to R10 a day for maintenance and food. When social workers eventually remove the children for placement, they do not give me the vouchers to claim back the money spent on the children whilst they were staying with me. That is a real problem, and yet we cannot leave these children without any support.

Mrs Mooi gave examples of children who had been left for a long time waiting for the district surgeon to examine them for evidence of rape. Over the Easter period many children were raped in Orange Farm. One of them was an 11 year old deaf girl who also could not speak. Her mother, a single parent, was a domestic worker and during her absence from home, a man repeatedly raped her daughter. He became so arrogant and nasty that one day he stayed until the mother came home and he told her that he and the girl were lovers. The mother and the neighbours asked him to communicate with the girl to prove that the relationship was based on mutual consent. This he could not do. When he realised the anger of the people he ran away. Mrs Mooi took the child to the police station:

> I was there from 8.00 p.m. to 3.00 a.m. and I could not get a single policeman to take a statement and arrange for the district surgeon to examine the child. One of them said they could not accuse an adult man

based on the evidence from a child because sometimes children imagine things. Another one said they do not have facilities to communicate with deaf and dumb people. They sat there, ignored my pleas and fell asleep. That child was left for 4 days without washing because the district surgeon had not examined her.

The community continued looking for the man. He in turn went to the police, claiming that the mother of this girl was organising people to kill him. Instead of finding out why the community wanted him, the police accepted his story and went to arrest the woman. Fortunately she was not in her house when they went for her. The community was angry because people believed and felt that the police were keen to respond to rapists' complaints but did nothing to investigate sexual assaults on women and children. Not surprisingly, women wanted to take the matter into their own hands and deal with the rapist themselves. This feeling is strengthened by the ease with which the courts allow rapists to be bailed thus offering them further opportunity to rape.

This desperation led to the killing of a man who raped an infant in a squatter camp and the castration of another man who had raped a young girl. Even women who do not agree with vigilante groups, like Mrs Mooi who manages the Luthando Centre, are irritated by the leniency shown to the rapists and believe that if women did kill the perpetrators, the government would not give bail to rapists.

Another 11 year old, raped by an old family 'friend' at knifepoint, was left for two weeks waiting to be examined. The combination of stale semen and vaginal bruising produced maggots. Delays do not only happen in Orange Farm. National television programmes on violence against women and children tell the same tale in other parts of the country. A middle-aged white woman reported a similar incidence when she was left for hours unwashed after a rape incidence. Eventually she went home and had a wash thus destroying any evidence for the court case. But many take the view that even if you stay unwashed and evidence is found, nothing seems to be done to rapists to deter them. If charged, they are released on bail and many continue to assault women and children. In some instances cases of rape are dismissed because the child's testimony is regarded either insufficient or inconsistent. In 1995 the Protea Magistrate's Court dismissed eight cases of rape on these grounds (Sowetan, 1995).

In another case in Orange Farm, a clergyman who had repeatedly raped a 12 year old girl was not convicted because the doctor's documentation of the case was lost from the court files. The suggestion that a detective was paid R2,000 to remove the file was never investigated.

Another distressing case known to Orange Farm is that of a white farmer who has been raping the children of his farm workers for years. One of them has a child from him. The six abused children were moved from the farm into the Centre whilst the case was investigated. The court found the farmer guilty. He was given six years but the people in Orange Farm say he is still in his house and suspect that he is out on bail.

The Luthando Centre is providing a vital service for children who have been abused. This offers valuable immediate post-incident intervention. What the South African community needs is a national solution. Taken individually or in their totality none of the presented explanations account for a sane, educated, professional man who is employed, living in a comfortable house with his wife, who rapes his four year old daughter. This man, holding his daughter in his arms because he could not disengage, was taken in an ambulance to a hospital where his wife worked as a nursing sister, to be separated from the child who was by then half unconscious from severe bleeding and pain. It is a national problem that awaits to be addressed not just by women but all agencies in the country.

Political Violence

Violence linked to political oppression has been the main feature of the apartheid regime. Attacks on children reached a horrendous climax in 1976 when thousands of black school children were gunned down by the police and the armed forces. The children were protesting and challenging the oppressive racist system encapsulated in the compulsory use of Afrikaans in education which the children identified as the oppressors' language. Hundreds of children were killed instantly. Some who were severely injured died later in hospitals. Others were maimed and remain paralysed and many who were not badly injured managed to escape and found refuge in neighbouring countries. Many stayed and continued the struggle.

The violence faced by children did not end with the demise of the apartheid system. It continued as an aftermath, affecting children in different ways. During the faction fights between black political groups engineered by the adherents of the Nationalist government, many children suffered untold violence (Truth and Reconciliation Commission). Some were killed with their families and others watched their relatives being killed. The violent climate continues to exist in some areas among such groups as drug 'pushers'. Some children live in areas which are dominated by gangsters whose lives revolve around drugs, drink and fights. Ewing, who spoke to five- year-olds who live in such areas concluded that:

> The environment in which many of our youngsters are growing up constitutes child abuse as clearly as physical or sexual assault (Ewing, 1996, p.15).

Their childhood is 'stolen' by violence. It is that violence which has made many vulnerable to mental illness.

Children and Mental Illness

For many years mental illness has been beset by controversy. The major dispute is over the concept of mental illness, its causation and what is actually meant by the assertion that a person is mentally ill (Torkington, 1991). Apart from my conviction that a social perspective gives scope for understanding mental illness, in South Africa a lot of emphasis is placed on the role of social factors in the causation of mental illness among black South African children. Such is the concern about social factors, in particular violence, that RECOVERY, a journal for Research and Cooperation On Violence, Education and Rehabilitation of Young people has been established as a forum to discuss the issues involved.

A major barrier in knowing the extent to which the mental state of children is affected by violence is the lack of reliable statistics. A study conducted by Irlam on childhood disability (two-nine years), which includes mental illness, in the KwaZulu-Natal Province, for example, offers a crude prevalence rate of 3.4 percent broken down as shown in the following Table (Irlam, 1996).

Table 4.2 Types of disabilities among children aged between two to nine years

Type of disability	Percentage
Hearing	29.9
Vision	21.6
Learning	14.4
Speech	11.3
Mental	8.2

Table 4.2 (continued)

Mobility	4.1
Fits	6.2
Developmental delay	4.1

As Desmond observes, these statistics do not appear to reflect the reality and the extent of social and economic experience whose consequences in terms of disability one would expect to be higher than what the above statistics suggest:

> This does not make too much sense to me. Presumably many children have more than one disability so the total should come to over 100 percent. I also suspect that many of the figures are too low. Given the degree of malnutrition, for, example, a lot more than 4.1 percent of 3.4 percent of the population must suffer developmental delay. I think it probable that the majority of two generations of Africans have been physically and/or mentally stunted because of poverty and malnutrition. (Private communication)

Expectations of higher figures of children psychologically affected by violence is also expressed by professionals who work with children. Ngesi, a Psychologist, for example, puts the figure of children affected by political violence in the KwaZulu-Natal at 26,790 and he states that if we add those children who have been physically, sexually and emotionally abused, the figure is much higher. Many children who have been affected by violence develop stress-related problems such as depression and post-traumatic stress disorders. These effects are reflected in children's drawings in schools. Similar kinds of drawings were produced by the many children who took part in the Truth and Reconciliation Commission (Ngesi, 1997).

Ngesi's assertion that many children who have been affected by violence develop mental health problems finds support in the study by Ensink and associates (1997) in Cape Town. The study investigated the extent to which children exposed to community violence develop Post Traumatic Stress Disorder (PTSD). The study was a cross section of 60 Xhosa speaking children with a high risk of past exposure to violence. The children aged 10-16 came from Khayelisha, a township outside Cape Town. 30 of the children came from a children's home and 30 from a school.

The results revealed that all the children had been exposed to violence, 56 percent had experienced violence and 95 percent had witnessed it. Forty five percent witnessed one or more killings whilst 55 percent witnessed one or more stabbing, shooting or other violent attack. Thirty three percent had at least seen one dead body, and 40 percent had heard gun shots. The children reported graphically the violent acts they had seen:

- a man hacked to death after shooting a woman;
- a man who was shot when he was kneeling down with arms up in a gesture of surrender;
- a gang fight in which 2 members had their heads hacked off;
- a man beaten to death with bricks by the community after he had slit a woman's throat.

All children had symptoms which suggested that their mental state had been negatively affected by the violence. These included:

> Recurrent recollections of the traumatic event (59), avoidance of thoughts and feelings associated with the event (51), poor sleep (46), restricted range of affect (43), and diminished interest and pleasure (Ensink et al, 1997, p.8).

Many of the children also suffered from irritability, distressing dreams, poor concentration, detachment from other people and a sense of a shortened future.

These findings echo the results of work by Killian and associates (1995) in Richmond, one of the areas worst hit by violence in the KwaZulu-Natal province. The stress-related symptoms in their study included nightmares, inability to concentrate, problems with memory, feeling sad all the time, feeling angry all the time, difficulty in falling asleep and spells of crying.

Other professionals who work with children note the aggressive behaviour displayed by five year olds who live in a violent environment. A teacher and community worker described the children with whom she worked:

> ... aggressive in play, in their dealing with each other. It has taken a year to get Brinton to relate properly to the other children. But what worries me most is their obsession with sex and their association of aggression with sex. It's not healthy for five-year-olds to be constantly talking about sex the way they do, not with innocent curiosity but in a blatant way, using graphic and violent language (Ewing, p.16).

What is of major concern to professionals, community groups and families is the absence of nationally endorsed provision for children suffering the effects of violence and the very limited service responses.

Mental Health Services for Children

In South Africa mental health services within the public sector are poor in general, and for children they are almost non-existent. A psychiatrist who has worked in all psychiatric hospitals in the Gauteng province stated that except for one hospital with ten beds, there are no admission beds for mentally ill children in most hospitals. Assessment, treatment and follow up is all done in day centres. A matron who works in one of the hospitals with clinics for children with mental illness explained how inappropriate such a provision is:

> They come in and they are handed drugs and they go home. By noon they have all gone. Some of them are very young people who should have some rehabilitation programmes. Many have been the victims of the political struggle, who, as children, witnessed the killing of their parents.
>
> There is one boy who was with his grandmother when they were attacked. The grandmother hid him in an empty beer calabash. The attackers came in and killed the grandmother and this boy saw and heard everything. When they left the boy came out and just ran away in the dark. He was eventually found the following day by the villagers who survived the attack. The grandmother was his only close relative. When he comes here they just give him drugs. Nobody has ever looked at that history, or asks why such a young boy needs these drugs.

It is this lack of effective and responsive services in the public sector which has prompted the development of community based facilities in the voluntary sector.

Community-based Mental Health Facilities

Two models of community based mental health services: The Empilweni Centre and the South Coast Hospice Trauma Counselling Network (SCHTCN) are the focus of this section.

Empilweni Centre (a Place of Health)

In its operation this Centre draws from traditional psychiatric provision. It was established by the Department of Psychiatry in the University of Cape Town in partnership with the community in Khayelisha. The project was set up in response to a request by the South African National Civic Organisation (SANCO), to provide a service for children who were presenting with problems, at school, within the family and in the community.

The children who use the Centre come with a wide range of traumatic experiences. They have been physically and/or sexually abused, exposed to violence and many have suffered from neglect. As a result many of them suffer from depression and anxiety, they struggle in their schoolwork and many become truants. Some of them have severe behavioural problems such as stealing, lying and fighting.

Referrals to the Centre come from schools, social workers, health visitors, hospitals and individual families. The 301 children who were using the facilities of the Centre at the time of my research ranged between six and sixteen years of age. Those who attended the Centre did so after school hours. For some children it was necessary to work with the whole family and for them, sessions were held in their own homes. In addition to individual and family counselling, the Centre had a boys' and a girls' group. The focus in both groups was on therapy and education. Children were introduced to life skills. They were encouraged to be assertive, to say what they thought and felt about what had happened to them. The secure and supportive environment of the Centre fostered an open trusting atmosphere within which experiences were shared. In that sharing they learnt to be sensitive and accepting of others' problems. In the boys' group for example, there were some children with learning disabilities. Members of the group were encouraged to be accepting of these children:

> We sometimes have drawing and painting workshops where we ask boys to do an image of a person or of themselves. When the children with learning disabilities paint something that does not resemble a person, nobody laughs at them or tells them that what they have painted is not a person. They are given support and encouragement. We promote an atmosphere in which the boys develop a sense of respect for themselves and others. We assist them in building communication with each other and with their families (Community mental health worker, 1997).

In addition to such activities, children were taken out on a variety of outings during weekends and school holidays. These excursions also served as vehicles for general education. When they went to Robben Island, for example, they learned about the history of the island in relation to President Mandela and the black struggle. That in turn led to the general history of South Africa to the present time. They were encouraged to look at that situation from different points of view and suggest what changes could be introduced, with what consequences and benefits.

Sport was another avenue that staff used to develop self-esteem and integration to the wider community. At the time of the research there was a move to create a soccer club which would be linked to other soccer clubs in the community:

> It is important that the children who come here are not isolated from the rest of the community. They should mingle and be in touch with other young people. We really need to unify the youth in Khayelisha, and a soccer team is the best way of doing this (Community mental health worker, 1997).

The girls' group did not appear to be as active. Attendance was erratic and even when girls had promised to come; they often failed to turn up. Staff thought there were a number of reasons for this:

> The girls are into boy friends and this rules them. They do not want to go to school. They drink, they smoke and they co-habit with men much older than they are because they give them money to buy fashionable clothes. We are constantly going to the teachers in schools asking them to take the girls back into classes, but quite often they fail to attend and they get thrown out again and again. These are young girls between 12 and 16 years old (Community mental health worker, 1997).

Staff also suggested that there might be other reasons why these girls went out with older men. Many of them had been sexually abused by a father or an uncle. This might have led them to believe that having sex with an older man was the norm. Others might have been searching for a father figure since many of them lived with single mothers.

The project had a team of six staff, one of whom was a qualified social worker. The other five were drawn from the community and trained as community mental health workers. This was to make sure that the project met its objective which was to provide a service, delivered by people who understood and were familiar with the local community they served:

> The main objective of this model is to empower ordinary citizens in the community to respond to problems which affect child and adolescent mental health - as far as possible, by building their capacity through education and skills training. The training of members of the community to lead and direct this process is central to this objective (Ensink et al, p63).

The team was holistic in its approach which enabled the provision of different aspects of needs presented by the children and the community served. The staff had to be able to identify children with neurological and deep psychiatric problems and refer them to relevant professionals, many of whom came to the Centre and worked on a voluntary basis. They had to have counselling skills for individuals, groups of children and family members. They had to be familiar with a number of educational topics which provided useful tools in building up the children's self esteem, identity and confidence. They had to be familiar with and understand the local community politics in order to be accepted in their interventionist role. They had to be aware that underlying the behaviour of the children was poverty and destitution which was reflected in the degree of malnutrition and illness in many of the children using the Centre. Their understanding of this link was reflected in staff's involvement in obtaining maintenance grants for families. The social worker, who supervised the team, encouraged this holistic approach because without it the project would have found it difficult to achieve its objectives because it would not have been fully embraced by the community.

The Empilweni Centre was highly regarded in the community not only for the work it did for children with mental health problems but also children with learning disabilities. Within a year of the Centre's life 26 children were assessed and found to be having learning disabilities. This information helped families to understand the behaviour of their children and enabled them to set realistic expectations in their school achievement. They were enabled to make appropriate educational placement with the help of the team.

People in the community made their appreciation known to the team when a positive change was evident in children who had been regarded as a 'problem' for their families or the community at large:

People will point to a child and say 'just look how that boy's behaviour has changed since he started attending the Centre, he is now very polite and considerate'. Some schools also report good progress after the boys start coming here (Community mental health worker, 1997).

The Centre was funded by non-governmental moneys. There was a hope that in future the government would take it over and provide main stream funding for the service. However, among those who are closely involved with the Centre, there was a concern that in the restructuring of mental health provision which was being undertaken, a Centre like Empilweni might be phased out. The concern was that the work the Centre did could not be done effectively within the proposed new structure:

> Reflected in the mental health policy of the new Government of South Africa is an emphasis on developing community projects around specific psychosocial issues. Even if primary health care mental health services were developed, it is likely that only the more severe psychiatric disorders would be identified and treated at clinics. Over-extended primary care clinic staff could not feasibly provide counselling for parents and families around psychosocial problems. These problems ideally need to be treated within a broader preventive primary health care approach which is oriented towards community development, rather than from within a clinic-centred approach based on the medical model, and focused on treating physical health problems (Ensink et al, 1994 p.63).

The South Coast Hospice Trauma Counselling Network (SCHTCN)

The network was set up in 1993 when members of the community in the South Coast region of KwaZulu-Natal, which was heavily hit by political violence, identified the psycho-social problems faced by the survivors of political and criminal violence and the need for their treatment and rehabilitation. In conjunction with the Department of Health, members of the community applied for funding from the National Peace Accord Trust to train hospice members and nurses in order to manage their own and their patients' stress and trauma. A one-year basic counselling skills training course was set up.

Like the Empilweni project, the course recruited people from the community who had no formal qualifications. In addition people with some form of qualification such as teachers, priests, police, nurses, hospice workers and many more were accepted for training. Two years after the course started 66 people qualified and of those 43 were recommended to work as lay counsellors.

The counsellors work as a network which stretches across towns, villages and rural areas. They usually use traditional trauma counselling methods for individuals and groups. Culturally based story telling, drawings, songs, poetry and for some, prayer, are all used in the counselling process. Rather than imposing or assuming shared understanding of the effects of trauma, counsellors encourage individuals and family groups to work with the meaning they attach to the traumatic experience and the effect it had on them. There is no general formula followed which disregard specific and individual needs. Sessions take place in settings which suit clients. This could be a person's family home, a hospice, a refugee camp or a hospital. Group sessions may take place in a community or a church hall, a school hall or a clinic. Public health education takes the form of talks in churches after the service, in schools and in clinics whilst patients are waiting to be seen.

From July 1996 to June 1997 lay counsellors worked with 1534 people. Referrals were by word of mouth as well as through health workers, teachers, women's groups and non-governmental organisations. The majority of cases were of sexual and domestic violence involving children. The most common victims of criminal and political violence were children under 18 years old.

In the evaluation of this project counsellors were asked what the people using the service said was the most useful aspect of the network:

> ...recognition and affirmation as an individual within a private and confidential setting...the person using the counselling process as an advocacy tool to facilitate easier and swifter networking and access to resources...relief through 'venting', and 'clarity' from 'guided' problem-solving (Stavrou, 1997, p.9).

In the course of their work lay counsellors face a lot of problems, the most common being feelings of anger and helplessness in the face of tremendous trauma inflicted on people, frustration because of limited skills which prevent them from in-depth work with children and families; lack of time and money to visit places inaccessible by car; and frustration because they are not recognised or respected by social workers and mental health professionals. One of the major recommendations by the lay counsellors was that the government and professional bodies, in particular, Nursing and Social Work Councils should recognise their work which was critical in the treatment and rehabilitation of trauma survivors:

The network structure facilitates a swift, crisis management response to referrals. Survivors of violence immediately need to have their safety and security needs met, as well as requiring urgent physical and psychological first aid. The network volunteers are able to work swiftly and make broad ranging independent referrals. High levels of motivation and community-based networking often overcome communication and transport problems, factors which often limit accessibility of state services (Stavrou, p.10).

Lay counsellors are, typically, members of the communities they serve. They are known, accepted and well respected within their communities. They are therefore more likely to know and be told about what goes on and are accorded legitimacy to act swiftly when a need arises. Most of them are highly politicised, socially aware people whose motivation in volunteering is to 'uplift the community and to develop the nation'. They view their trauma support work as an opportunity to 'live out their social politics as opposed to party political views' (Stavrou, p.10).

Reflection In this chapter I have presented a disturbing picture of the violence and its mental health consequences experienced by children in South Africa. In the process of coping with the aftermath of that experience, lessons have emerged which have significant implications for both training and practice in social work in South Africa. These lessons are expressed in the following requirements.

- a holistic approach, not only in training but also in practice for all those working with traumatised children;
- a robust partnership with local communities served;
- a flexibility in the attitude of professionally trained workers which enable an equal working relationship with communities served;
- a recognition of the expertise of community-based workers;
- an intervention that is culturally credible to different groups served;
- to revisit the origins of places such as Philani, the Luthando Centre and the Empilweni Centre – establish whether there are other such hopeful and people-driven places – and work with their Directors, staff and young people to explore and test out different solutions to very long standing problems;
- national leadership and policy to pursue actively the goal of mental health improvement for all.

References

Campbell, C. (1996), 'Social Identity and Violence in the domestic and political sphere: a gender common denominator'?, In Glanz E. and Spiegal, Andrew D. (ed) *Violence and Family Life in Contemporary South Africa: Research and Policy Issues,* Human Science Research Council.

Cape Times, 16 July (1997).

Corby, B. (1994), *Child Abuse - Towards a Knowledge Base,* Open University Press.

Department of Health (1995), *Annual Report.*

Desmond, C. (ed) (1977), 'Research and Co-operation on Violence, Education and Rehabilitation of Young People', *Recovery,* January/February, vol.1, No.9/10, p.13.

Ensink, K., Robertson, B., Zissis, C. and Leger, P. (1997), *Postraumatic Stress Disorder in Children Exposed to Violence,* unpublished paper.

Ensink, K. and Richardson, K.A. (1994), 'The Empilweni Project', *South African Journal of Child Adolescent Psychiatry,* vol.6, No.2, p 63.

Ewing, D. (1996), 'Where Childhood is Stolen by Violence', *Recovery,* vol.1, No.8, November/December, p.15.

Henderson, P. (1996), 'Communication and Corporal Punishment. Beatings as a Standard Form of Admonishing Children in New Crossroads Households' in Glanz, E. and Spiegal, Andrew D. (ed) *Violence and Family Life in Contemporary South Africa: Research and Policy Issues,* Human Science Research Council.

Irlam, J. (1996), *A Rural Childhood Prevalence Study in KwaZulu-Natal,* unpublished report, Amatikulu Primary Health Care Centre, KwaZulu-Natal.

Kempe, C., Silverman, F., Steele, B., Droegemueller, W. and Silver, H. (1962), 'The Battered Child Syndrome', *Journal of the American Medical Association,* 181, pp.17-24.

Killian, B.J., Higson-Smith, R.C. and Govender, K. (1995), *The Effects of Chronic Violence On Children Living in South African Townships,* unpublished research report.

Lund Committee (1996), *Report of the Lund Committee on Child and Family Support,* August, South Africa.

Magidela, T. (1996), 'Mothers Start to speak the Unspeakable', *Recovery,* November/December, vol.1, No.8, p.22.

McKerrow, N. (1996), 'Spread of HIV linked to increase in sexual abuse', *Recovery,* November/December, vol.1, p.5.

Ngesi, J. (1997), 'School Psychologists', *Recovery,* August/September, vol.2, No.13.

Patel, L. (1993), *Children and Women in South Africa: A Situational Analysis,* UNICEF and the National Children's Rights Committee.

Ramphele, M. (1996), 'How sweet is Home? Family Dynamics in New Crossroads', in Glanz and Speigal, *op cit.*

Sowetan, 1 December 1995.

Sowetan, 6 March 1995.

Stavrou, V. (1997), 'Volunteers Key to Survival Care', *Recovery,* August/September, vol.2, No.13, p.8.

Straus, M. and Gelles, R. (1980), *Behind Closed Doors, Violence in the American Family,* Anchor Press, New York.

Torkington, N.P.K. (1991), *Black Health - a Political Issue,* Catholic Association for Racial Justice and Liverpool Institute of Higher Education.

Waldby, C., Clancy, A., Emetchi, J. and Summerfield, C. (1989), 'Theoretical perspectives on father-daughter incest' in Driver, E. and Broisen, A. (eds), *Child Sexual Abuse - Feminist Perspectives,* MacMillan, p.102.

5   Women and Health

There is no shortage of feminist literature analysing the historical position of women. The long-standing patriarchal domination that has faced women has left us invisible in almost all aspects of historical development. There is no accepted historical record of female popes, bishops and priests, no revered female equivalent of Leonardo da Vinci or Beethoven. We have founding fathers but no founding mothers of Sociology, History, Philosophy or Medicine. Feminists argue that this is not because women were incapable but because they were generally incapacitated and discriminated against so that some outstanding female creativity was subsumed under male achievements, or erased from 'his-story'. Latterly, 'her-story' is gaining ground and some achievements and the processes by which women's endeavours were diminished are coming to light. For black women, diminishment was the function of oppression based on gender, race and class. As Margaret Walker observed:

> We have an ongoing struggle for the rights of Black people, and we have never lost sight of the fact that we are women, exploited as much because of our sex as because of our race and poverty (Sterling, 1988, p.xi).

In apartheid South Africa oppression was served by traditional patriarchy and was rigorously maintained by legislation which proffered black women the status of 'perpetual minors'. Section 11 (3) of the South African Bantu Administration Act No. 38 of 1927, Sub-section (b) reads:

> A Bantu woman who is a partner in a customary union, and who is living with her husband, shall be deemed to be a minor and her husband shall be deemed to be her guardian (United Nations, 1978).

In the Natal province the operation of Section 27 (2) of the Natal Code of Law No. 46 of 1887 stated that unless emancipated, an African woman remained a perpetual minor under the guardianship of a man – her father or his heir, her husband or his heir. Emancipation was dependent upon being single, proof that the woman owned immovable property, was of good character, educated and had thrifty habits. A married woman never qualified for emancipation even when she was deserted or unsupported by her husband.

As a minor, a woman could not, in her own right, enter into any contract, sue or be sued and could not own property except her own personal effects. She could neither travel nor be employed without the consent of her male guardian. Legally, for all practical purposes, there was nothing a black woman could do unless the man under whose charge she was deemed to be, had given his permission. This legally enforced patriarchy was strengthened by the Pass Laws which disqualified women from urban residency if they could not prove that they had lived in the area legally for a stipulated period. In Cape Town, for example, women who could not prove that they had lived there for 15 years were 'endorsed out' to a rural area if they became unemployed or widowed. Personal experience of these laws will illuminate how restrictive they were. I was born in Natal and therefore destined to be a perpetual minor. When I went to train as a nurse in the Cape Province I had to have my father's permission. Soon after finishing training, I was offered a three month job in another hospital in the same province. Within a month of starting work, I was summoned to the Local Government's Bantu Administrative Office and was instructed to leave the province within 72 hours because I had no legal right to be in that province. The hospital desperately needed my services because the nurse I was replacing was still ill. The white hospital superintendent intervened, and I remained there until the member of staff I was replacing was well enough to resume work.

My second experience arose when I was accepted for work in a hospital in Natal, my own province. I needed accommodation in the local township. When I approached the relevant administrative office the white officer looked me over and said:

> We have no control over who the hospital employs. We have no accommodation for you here. As far as we are concerned you can sleep in the gutter. But what we do require from you as soon as possible, if you want to avoid prison, is a written letter from your father giving you permission to be here.

When I decided to come and study in England the forms to get a passport had to be signed by my father. Without his permission I would have never left South Africa.

These laws were not as purposeless as they appear. The success of the capitalist system depended on a network of apartheid laws which ensured that the majority of black women remained in rural areas for the reasons outlined by Wolpe. While legally that system is gone, its framework has not been fully dismantled and many black women remain caught and continue to suffer from the consequences.

Women and Poverty

In South Africa poverty and the unequal distribution of health services had undermined the health and wellbeing of many black people Within that general picture it is women and children whose health has been severely eroded. That erosion has been more marked in rural areas where women, children, elderly people, the unemployed and the sick, regarded as 'superfluous appendages' in urban areas, were dumped, thus swelling the numbers of the already crowded 13 percent land space reserved for Africans by the 1913 Land Act. A characteristic common to all rural areas is unemployment. This, coupled with a continuing decline in rural agricultural production, has led to abject poverty with pervasive health challenges, particularly for women and children. These begin before birth:

> ...with poor maternal nutrition contributing to prematurity and low birth weight. During childhood, poor nutrition inhibits normal growth and development, lack of hygienic facilities predisposes to infestations with scabies, head lice and intestinal worms... (Blane, 1991, p.114).

As mothers, housewives and carers, women are constantly struggling to make ends meet. It is not unusual for women to eat less or nothing at all when there is not enough food, in order to ensure that the husband and then the children have sufficient to eat. Not only is she expected to cook the food, but also to find what to cook. The family expects this and she expects it of herself. In the minority of families where husbands work and send money home the situation is not critical. But in the village where some of this research was done, many women are widows, there is no widow's pension, and many men are unemployed. Some women undertake jobs such as fetching water or firewood for which they are paid small amounts of money or a dish of mealies, beans or nuts. For long term survival some women help in weeding the fields with an agreement that they will be paid in food when the produce is ripe.

The poverty for some women is so great that many bear the tangible signs of deficiency diseases. The most affected are women of child-bearing age because of the specific nutritional needs during pregnancy and the lactation period. Various studies carried out from the 1970s onwards show how such women did not only have below minimum energy levels but also suffered from iron deficiency anaemia. A study of ante-natal women in one area in KwaZulu-Natal showed that one third of the women were anaemic and two thirds lacked folate, a vitamin B complex found in leafy vegetables. The combination of poor nutrition and lack of health services for black women is reflected in the differential maternal mortality rates per 100,000 live births per annum which in 1992 was 58 for Africans, 22 for coloureds, 8 for whites and 5 for Indians (Finchman *et al*, 1993). Once again these figures underestimate the number of black women who die during childbirth because they exclude women in rural areas where 55 percent of the total black female population lived.

The economic status of all women has not changed much in the 1990s. Their participation in the labour market has increased but it is still only 40 percent of the labour force. Financially, few of those who are employed benefit. The 1991 census revealed that women accounted for only 9 percent of the people who had an annual income of R300,000 or more and 59 percent of those whose income ranged between R1 and R999. The low pay of black women reflects their employment domains and opportunities. 30 percent are domestic workers. As directors in major South African companies, black women account for 0.5 percent. Whilst a large proportion of women are employed in textile, clothing and leather industries, the majority are self-employed in what Lund (1996) calls the 'survivalist' or 'for own account' sector.

Many women in the 'survivalist' sector spend the whole day sitting on city centre pavements selling fruit – oranges, pears, apples, bananas – piled in groups of four or five at prices that undercut nearby supermarkets. In areas like the beach front in Durban, where the goods sold are mainly curios imported from other African countries, women sleep alongside their goods. The majority are from rural areas and they bring blankets and their babies if they are breast feeding. They spend weeks on the beach front and only go home to take money to the family. Many do not have money to buy directly from producers and they are therefore employed by those who have. One woman was being paid R300 a month. In addition to this financial exploitation, women working in this sector face threats of being robbed or attacked as well as harassment from a wide range of officials with whom they have to negotiate in the process of selling their goods. These are the concerns which led to the establishment of the Self-Employed Women's Union (SEWU). I visited the SEWU office in Durban and interviewed the organiser.

SEWU started in 1994 and was the first union for women. All the employees had worked for recognised unions. For 12 years the organiser was a shop steward with the South African Clothing and Textile Union and later became the Vice Chairperson of the Council of South African Trade Unions (COSATU) in the Natal region. Their union experiences gave them insight into women's marginalisation and disempowerment.

- the joining fee is R10 and the monthly subscription fee is R5. For this the Union provides a number of services.
- it builds unity between women whose work is not recognised;
- develops negotiating skills so that women can negotiate directly with the City Council, police, small contractors and middle-men, civil and political organisations through their own representatives;
- assists women with legal advice;
- assists women in solving problems, such as child care, credit, lack of maternity, and sick or disability benefits;
- develops lobbying skills so that women can organise to get laws changed if they are not suitable to their needs;
- develops leadership skills among women who are self-employed;
- provides access for women to other organisations which offer facilities such as skills training, credit and loan facilities, legal assistance, health advice, assistance and relief or counselling for survivors of violent attacks, including rape.

There are three offices, two in KwaZulu-Natal and one in the Western Cape. The aim is to develop a network of offices in South Africa providing assistance to women who are self-employed. A group of women that the union has had difficulty in reaching is that of prostitutes. As the organiser noted:

> These are our children and we must assist them. The work they do is dangerous. Not only are they in danger of being raped, robbed, stabbed or killed, but they can also be infected by HIV. They have no links with medical or any form of health resources. They need support whilst they work as prostitutes but we also need to help those who want to stop by providing training for other jobs.

This discussion prompted me to look at this oldest of occupations.

Women and Prostitution

Prior to going to South Africa, I had been involved with colleagues on a study of prostitution in Liverpool. I was therefore interested to discover if there were similarities between the experiences of women in Liverpool and South Africa. I met three women: Jane, who owned a house used by seamen and prostitutes in the 1980s and 1990s in Durban, and Janice and Jean in Cape Town. Jane drew my attention to the changes in the pattern and the people involved in prostitution:

> I sold liquor to seamen who used to dock in Durban. I had a big lounge and the women and the seamen would come and have a drink together. The men would choose the women they wanted. Some took the women back to their ship, others went to hotels and some used rooms in the house. It was all very civilised. We all got to know each other well. Sometimes the seamen would pay me to cook food and we would all have a party. On most occasions the men would take their partners to the movies or dance clubs and generally give them a good time.

Many of the men used to return to the same women with whom they corresponded after leaving the docks. Some of them used to send money to their partners and bring presents for their children.

Jane's responsibility extended to the health of both men and women:

> I knew that the seamen were clean because they are checked by a doctor before they get a job, and also when they are in the company's employment. So I used to make sure that the girls were also clean. If any of them was infected, I used to get some injections for them.

I asked Jane what her understanding was of men's use of prostitutes. The case for seamen was clear in so far as they were away from their wives and girl friends. The reasons for men who were not sailors included:

- men looking for fun through sexual activities which they thought they could not have with their wives;
- men whose wives were unfaithful and as a result their relationship had broken down;
- men who liked a variety of sexual partners;
- 'kinky' men whose sexual satisfaction embraced:
  - wearing women's underwear;
  - watching women having sex;

- watching two men having sex with one woman at the same time;
- watching other people having sex;
- wanting to be tied up and beaten up.

A white man used to take women to his house and ask them to lie for two hours in a coffin whilst he sat and watched them.

Thus prostitution is not just about sexual intercourse but a whole range of practices for which men are prepared to pay.

I asked Jane why women entered prostitution. Many of them came from broken homes and violent families. Some became pregnant early in life and had to earn a living as single parents. Others were married women who came out occasionally to earn money for the family. In some cases husbands knew about this. Many of them had been in children's homes. The driving force was money. This was confirmed by Janice from Cape Town:

> I have a boy aged four years. I am a single mother and I have no job. There are just no jobs for us here. I only come out three times a week to earn money for rent and to feed my child. If there was a job I would take it.

Janice lives with her partner who looks after the child whilst she is out working. Did she feel that she was being exploited?

> No, I don't. When we met I was not working and he was. He looked after me and my baby. Now he is not well and I think it is only fair that I should provide for him. If I did not work we would be homeless and there is no way I will do that to my child.

Jean who looked 12, even though she assured me she was 14 years old, entered prostitution through her friendship with other young women.

> I had a boyfriend and one day when we were on our own he said let us try it. When I told my friends that we have had a go they said I should come with them and try it out with other men. I didn't like doing it at first, but I don't mind it now. They pay me good money.

Good money was R80 when the norm for most women was R60. Jean knew why she was being paid higher than other women:

> It is because I am young. When I am standing with other women men will ask me to go with them. Usually it is white men who pick me up and

take me to their flats. I do anything they want me to do as long as they pay me.

Jean makes a lot of money with which she buys a lot of expensive clothes. She tells her parents that her boyfriend buys them for her and tells the boyfriend that her parents buy them. Neither party question her lie.

Jane believes the dangers facing South African men and women have intensified. As a result of political unrest, many parents have been killed, leaving a lot of children with no means of survival. Many children have entered prostitution. If they are offered jobs they get low pay because they have no qualifications. Male managers were reported to have sex with them before offering them a job, and during the employment period, and if they refuse, they get dismissed. For many, prostitution offers high wages and independence. Drug abuse has drawn prostitution into a complex cycle of criminal activities. The need for money to buy drugs means that women, particularly young women, have unprotected sex and work with pimps who are also involved in drugs and other criminal activities including robbing punters.

The sex workers' experience in South Africa is determined by the colour of their skin and their economic position. In general white prostitutes do not appear to face the same problems. Since the end of apartheid, which kept prostitution under wraps, an increasing number of upmarket 'entertainment centres' have sprung up in city centres. Advertisements accompanied by scantily dressed women, dominate the classified advertising sections of mainstream newspapers and leave readers in no doubt as to what is on offer. For example, an advertisement stated that a private and discreet upmarket salon offered 'a 100 percent satisfaction paradise through the availability of stunning sexy ladies for erotic massages, lingerie shows, fantastic duo shows and escort services' (Cape Times, 1997).

The names of the rooms in these salons are equally explicit about the functions they do – Deep Throat Dome, Porn Palace, Pleasure Dome, Opulent New Venue and House of Lords.

Andrew Malone, of the London Sunday Times, visited one such centre, a former farmhouse converted into a palatial brothel. Some 40 women were relaxing at the bar before their shift started. The clients were mainly white middle-aged and wealthy men paying an entrance fee of R300 which did not include fees for services rendered by the women. As one client stated, these men regarded prostitution as a bit of fun:

It is just a bit of fun. Life is not as it used to be. We face the daily threat of crime and difficulty getting work as the government tries to put blacks in our jobs. It's a way of easing stress. Nobody gets hurt and the girls get paid well (Cape Times, 1997).

For women however, it is a question of survival. One of the women was a 21 year old student who worked at the centre to pay for her education. She confirmed that women working in these centres do not face the same dangers as those who work on the streets:

Here there is no chance of being robbed by pimps who control the trade on the streets. Here there are security guards. We also always use condoms (Cape Times, 1997).

Malone believes that the government shows no inclination to curb the sex industry:

However, the government has shown no inclination to launch a crackdown. Instead, it is promoting a new way to combat sex crime. Masturbate! Don't rape! Is the slogan of an official campaign. The other word for masturbation is Arm Struggle, a government newsletter says. 'Join the Arm Struggle and stop raping our mothers, our wives, sisters and children'. Guests at the Ranch were unimpressed by the campaign. 'Why bother when you can get somebody to do it?' winked Geoff, 45, a publisher, before disappearing into the Deep Throat Dome' (Cape Times, 1997).

Should the government crackdown on prostitution? What form will that crackdown take? Will it take into account and tackle the causes which push women into prostitution?

On 15 December 1995 South Africa ratified the United Nations Convention on the Elimination of All Forms of Discrimination Against Women. Within that acceptance the government has to make sure that women are not treated like objects that can be bought and sold, and it must make sure that women are not exploited as prostitutes. The Task Team charged with the task of exploring contentious issues around prostitution was guided by the terms of this Convention.

In 1996 the Gauteng Cabinet Committee on Safety and Security and Quality of Life mandated the Gauteng Ministry of Safety and Security to draft a policy and provide the Cabinet with statistics on sex work. Following a multi-agency two-day workshop, a Task Team was set up to explore and advise on issues surrounding prostitution. The recommendations of the Task Team have been widely supported. The Gauteng Cabinet, the Western Cape Province, the South African Human Rights Commission, and the Ministers of Welfare, Safety and Security and Justice are all in favour of decriminalisation of sex work. As a result the policing of sex work has been de-prioritised and instead of arresting sex workers police are now concentrating on protecting them from crime and violence.

A major focus of the law is on child prostitution. The police and the local government in Gauteng are targeting brothels which allow children under 18 years to work as prostitutes. The Minister of Safety and Security, the Human Rights Commission and the Gender Commission are also seeking to decriminalise same sex relationships. However, South Africa is a very conservative country. Some NGOs, churches and political parties are opposed to the direction taken by the government. This opposition will not however, stop the process which is based on the Human Rights Constitution. The Task Team has consulted with sex workers not only to encourage them to exercise their human rights but also to take part in a massive public education campaign which will lead to the establishment of a South African Sex Workers Collective.

The Task Team has also made a number of recommendations.

- 'child prostitutes' should be decriminalised and 'child prostitution' which is unacceptable should be criminally sanctioned;
- children and adults should be protected from trafficking within and across borders and those involved in trafficking be penalised;
- the pimp category should be redefined since people 'who live on the proceeds' include sex-workers' dependants – children, parents and partners/husbands, to ensure that the focus is on the exploitative nature of pimping and not on the person who benefits from the proceeds;
- sex work should be decriminalised and there should be no mandatory testing for sexually transmitted diseases, including HIV, on the basis that it is an unfair discrimination against sex workers. It breaches sexual workers' rights to equality and affronts their dignity, it is contrary to the spirit of the constitution and the notion of an open society based on democratic values, social justice, equality and fundamental human rights. Besides, as women tested today can get infected tomorrow, testing offers no guarantee that women will be free from infection;
- there should be no enforcement of safe sex, instead the focus should be on behaviour rather than on persons;

- there should be no registration or licensing of sex workers and sex workers should be provided with viable and realistic options to leave the industry.

The Task Team was not in favour of creating tolerance zones:

> Sex workers are a heterogeneous group both men and women, extending across all racial, cultural, sexual, financial and geographical boundaries. Similarly, those who avail themselves of the services provided by sex workers, the clientele, are to be found in all sectors of society. Moreover, sex work has de facto zoned itself. Brothels are found in certain parts of cities, towns and township centres. Similarly, sex workers who operate from the streets are found in some streets and not all streets. Moreover, it is inconceivable to force sex workers in affluent, upmarket places to operate in down-town places like Hillbrow (Radgoadi, 1997).

Like mandatory testing, the zoning of sex work would restrict sex workers' rights to choose where to trade, be difficult to enforce and therefore ineffective and costly and would drive sex workers into clandestine operation.

In countries like Holland, where tolerance zones have been established, and in those like Britain, where their establishment has been explored, the impetus came from the need to respond to residents' action groups and individuals who opposed prostitution when it impacted on their lives. In Liverpool for example, our study was a response to residents' complaints about the effects of prostitution which included an increase in criminal activities in the area and a wide range of 'nuisances' such as noise, litter, traffic, harassment of male and female residents, intimidation, drugs and associated crime as well as a bad reputation for the area. Another concern was the effect prostitution had on children, e.g. children getting to know about sex as a commercial commodity and the position of women within that industry at an early age. As one resident pointed out, this does not give children good models:

> It just didn't bother me or Sue until we had the kids. When the kids started growing up and started noticing things it became a problem and I started to resent it. When I was picking the kids up from school I'd be stopped and asked for a cigarette and business. Then one day I just got really pissed off and said to this woman, 'I live here, just leave me alone'. You do worry about what they will find or what they will see.

Another resident expressed the same concern about the children:

> I try to give her (daughter) positive role models and then she sees women selling themselves on the streets (Campbell et al, 1996, p.26).

In its recommendations the Task Team does not concern itself with the impact of prostitution on residents. It would be interesting and indeed very helpful for countries which have resorted to, and for those which are contemplating the establishment of tolerance zones, to know whether South Africa has experience of the conflicts described, and if it has, how it is dealing with these.

The development of tolerance zones has not always considered the needs of women. For example, the location of the zone in Amsterdam was not favoured by prostitute organisations. Some prostitute organisations are fundamentally opposed to such zones:

> ...they argue that they can reinforce the marginal pariah status of prostitutes. They also argue that some women will resist working in such regulated areas and will still opt for the streets (Campbell et al, p.146).

Contrary to expectations of a crack down, the government in South Africa is looking at prostitution in a way that acknowledges the human rights of prostitutes in the context of the democratisation of the country, and the path taken offers lessons for many countries that have to deal with prostitution.

Whilst all women involved in the sex industry face physical and health dangers, the colour of the women mediate the degree and the nature of that danger. Black women are not only in danger of being robbed or killed when they work on the streets, they have no supporting structures like those available to white women in these centres. Many of them, Jane informed us, come from townships and rural areas. Lack of transport means that they work through the night or sleep in the open until morning. Some are fortunate to have friends with flats. Others have friends who are caretakers who secretly let them sleep in the cleaning or store rooms of firms for which they work. This makes prostitution one of the most health undermining occupations for black women. Even for those who work in the townships, life is less safe than it is for white women working in the affluent centres (Malone, 1997).

Women and HIV/AIDS

The Task Team's reluctance to recommend mandatory testing for sex workers was based on the recognition that most women are in danger of contracting HIV. Their decision finds support in studies which have found low rates of infection among street prostitutes (EUROPAP, 1994). In the Liverpool study, health professionals and drug workers echoed a similar message but expressed concerns about the rising rates of other sexually transmitted diseases from non-paying partners such as chlamydia, and Hepatitis B and C. Excluding women who are drug injecting or have partners who inject, most prostitutes are familiar with safe practices which ensure that they are not exposed to HIV infection. On the whole it is external pressures such as police harassment, poverty and threats of violence which make it difficult for women to negotiate safe sex (Faugier *et al*, 1992). In South Africa black prostitutes share with the majority of black women pressures which arise from their position as women in a patriarchally dominated culture.

Social and Psychological Factors

Irrespective of their class position, black women tend not to have access to information. In rural areas for example, many women are illiterate and even those who can read have no access to newspapers or leaflets about the virus and its transmission. As a result there are a lot of myths and beliefs that the disease can be cured. Further, women's heavy workload leaves little time for them to worry about HIV.

In urban areas similar workloads arising from gender roles leave women little time to read, as the HIV/AIDS Regional Director explained:

> Both husband and wife work, but when they get home the husband sits down and reads the newspaper whilst the wife does all the housework when the domestic helper is off.

Women feel guilty if they do not fulfil their domestic roles. There is a tension between the demands of their role as professional workers and as housewives with unending responsibilities. Zola Njongwe, a superintendent at Pretoria Academic Hospital, explained how the 'juggling act' affected her:

> I've always had so many distractions. Women in South Africa tend to finish their basic degrees and then encounter problems if they want to do

post-graduate work after marriage because of their husbands and children. I remember studying late for an exam with a group of people. When I came home I found myself locked out of the house. He didn't understand what was the big deal (about studies). Men don't understand why home and kids are not enough. That's why women give up, they fear that they could lose it all. The compromise can be very painful (Health Systems Trust, 1998, p.7).

In this study we have come across women who have had similar experiences with their husbands who have used their dominant and culturally accepted positions of power to stop their wives seeking further education. One nursing sister described how her husband intervened in her studies:

A group of us started a part-time degree in nursing. We used to meet in each other's houses after work, maybe once a fortnight around the time when our assignments were due. He objected to me going out and said he did not want his wife going out in the dark. If that was a safety concern he could have given me a lift, we had a car. Besides, he never worried about me coming home in the dark from work. He never offered to pick me up. His objection had nothing to do with his concern for the safety of his wife, it was about me studying. To make sure I did not have help, he forbade my colleagues coming to our house for study.

Life was really becoming difficult. He was not just sleeping with other women, he had a child with one of them even though he denied this to me. But I knew it to be true because relatives of the woman told me. At home he was beating me and kicking me about over very minor arguments. On many occasions he sat talking to no one, even the kids were feeling the strain and they were not safe from his beatings. He used to start the arguments when we were in bed. One day he locked the door and hit me around the head, my nose started bleeding and he kicked me and told me not to dirty his carpet with blood, I should go to the bathroom and bleed there. When I went to see the doctor the following day he told me that I had a freshly burst eardrum.

Such appalling stress weakens women, challenges personal resources and undermines their resistance. I was told that when such women are infected with HIV they tend to develop AIDS and die more quickly than their partners.

Social Education for Married Life

In South Africa before marriage a bride-to-be is counselled by older women. She learns that she should respect every member of her husband's household but above all, her husband in everything he says and does. More importantly, and more relevant to the virus, she must be sexually available to her husband, even when she knows that he sleeps with other women, or men for that matter. The Regional Director of HIV/AIDS explained:

> Women sleep with husbands knowing that they have a sexually transmitted disease, and that he sleeps with other women, because they are taught to accept sex with their husbands whatever the situation. Other people say 'oh, he has built a house for you, he gives you money, so what is your problem?' So, many women find themselves staying in abusive and health threatening situations. Even their own parents will tell them to go back to their husbands because, 'whoever said marriage was easy'.

Economic Pressure and Lack of Confidence

Some women, particularly young women, get involved in sex for financial reasons. Many women sell sex because they are desperate. The Regional Director knew a woman who had two children in the university and one in primary education. Her husband was an alcoholic and she went out at night to work in order to pay the education fees and to keep the family together. Some women are known to have had sex with a person who promises to pay for their education.

When women look for jobs, the men who appoint them may want sex in return. Some of these men do not use condoms. The women are not socialised in ways of assertion and do not say 'no'. That they are desperate for paid employment renders them especially vulnerable. Even school children are not immune. In some schools, the Regional Director stated, girls may compete with women teachers for 'love affairs' with male teachers. Schoolgirls have neither the confidence nor knowledge to say 'no' to a teacher who does not want to use a condom.

AIDS workers are concerned by the propensity for young girls to get pregnant at a very young age:

> Some young men seem keen to use condoms. Even now as I came to this meeting, they recognised the bag and knew that I was carrying condoms, so they shouted that they wanted some. But when you talk to the young men they say that girls do not want to use condoms. It looks as if the

girls want to become pregnant, and condoms stop them falling pregnant. But of course in the process they become infected with the virus.

The fact that some women do not use any form of contraceptive, and get infected by the virus, was confirmed by the prevalence of teenage pregnancies and by midwives:

> We get them from 12 years old. Some of them are so little they cannot deliver without a caesarean section. It is then that the AIDS virus reveals itself. The suture line just does not heal and when tests are done we then find out that the young girl is HIV positive.

The seventh in a series of national annual HIV surveys of women attending ante-natal clinics of public health services took place during October and November of 1996. It confirmed that it is the younger women who are mainly infected by the virus. Women in their twenties had the highest rates of infection at 17.5 percent and 15 percent for the 20-24 and 25-29 respectively. The report notes:

> Of particular concern are the pregnant women under twenty where a prevalence rate of 12.78 percent was found. Pregnancies at such a young age are often unplanned and might be a reflection of a group who is experimenting with sex. It seems reasonable therefore, to regard those teenagers who become pregnant as being a particular sub-set of their general age cohort, which is at increased risk of contracting HIV. It can then be argued that they are not representative of this age interval. On the other hand, this group reflects the most recent infections as this group also represents the age at which sexual activity starts (Doyle and Muhr, 1997, p.10).

There are obviously other reasons why young girls get pregnant, not least the pressures put on them by the un-negotiated norms in sexual behaviour. Culturally, women are not expected to take the initiative in sexual matters. Teenage girls will not seek advice about safe sex. Even when they reach adulthood they are embarrassed by sexual topics. In South Africa a woman is a woman if she can produce children. This offers one slant on their 'reluctance' to use condoms. It is known that young men will use the carrot of marriage, which is unlikely to materialise once the young woman is pregnant.

Another factor which weakens the fight against the virus is that young people are not confronted with the reality of AIDS. As an AIDS worker observed, this makes prevention very difficult:

This is a real problem in a number of ways. Firstly, a young person may have been told that he/she has AIDS, but the patient may not tell the parents who then spend a lot of money on traditional healers in the belief that the young person is suffering from a condition that Western medicine cannot cure. Secondly, the young person may not even tell his/her friends that he/she has AIDS. As a result young people may know about AIDS but they are not confronted with their own friends who have the disease, so for them, the problem remains theoretical, something with which adults frighten them. There is almost an unwritten law not to mention that people have died of AIDS. When prominent figures in the media die of AIDS nobody wants to say that the patient had AIDS. In this way people are not confronted with real people who have died of the disease.

What can be Done to Empower Women?

A whole range of measures are in place to tackle the increasing spread of infection in South Africa. The following summary outlines key messages suggested in seminars I attended which were aimed at empowering women.

Tackling Wider Issues of Inequality

Although the laws of apartheid which subjugated women to men have gone, custom and practice leaves women on the margins of equality. They do not, for example, inherit a title or property within their own families and their male siblings are regarded as the rightful inheritors. Society accepts this practice. Women do not yet feel that they matter in society. Such inequality gives rise to the morality which allows men to have as many sexual experiences as they choose. This licence is not extended to their wives who may be infected by their husbands to whom they cannot deny sex (Kelly, 1998).

Life Skills

Teaching children to say 'no' at a very early age to people who touch their bodies in ways that are wrong is a pressing need. There should be identifiable people who teach children about sexual behaviour from childhood onwards, not just about sexual activity but acceptable and non-acceptable behaviour. They must know how people should behave towards them. How this education might be undertaken merits careful thought if children are to give valued self images. Campaigns aimed at protecting children from sexual abuse would have to parallel assertion skills for children with focused and information-rich messages for mothers, boys and men. In a seminar on sexual rights and AIDS, I asked about the possibility of resurrecting time-honoured traditions as part of the fight against the AIDS epidemic.

Traditionally young people were taught when, where, and how to have sex. In the love life of a young woman there were a number of stages which were carefully monitored by older sisters, not necessarily siblings, but women from the same kinship group. In describing these stages I cannot speak for the whole of Africa but only of South Africa. The stages are part of the system within which I was brought up even though I did not take part in the rituals because by the time I reached mid-teens I was already in a boarding school and heavily influenced by Western culture and the practice itself was in decline.

The initial stage starts when the young girl is in her mid teens and she is approached by a suitor who declares his love for her. He pursues her wherever he can – he waits for her when she goes to fetch water from the river, when she goes for firewood, going to the shop or going to church. It is an accepted ritual that the man asks difficult questions and the young woman tries to answer them. If she fails the man can claim to have won, not just the quiz/argument but her love as well. He can then tell her sisters that he has won and they should give permission for the two to be lovers. The woman may not accept this. Even if the young woman fell in love with the suitor on the first day of his proposal, it is poorly regard to accept him immediately. It takes at least six months before the girl acquiesces. The longer the time, the better the girl is thought of by everyone in the community, including her suitor.

The couple adhere to regulations governing the relationship at this stage. They can be together as long as there are other people around, not necessarily with them, but near enough to ensure that they are not tempted to engage in any form of sexual activity. They must never be alone together after sunset.

In the next stage the man asks permission from her sisters for sexual rights. He pursues them with the same vigour he pursued the young woman. They tell him to go away because their sister is still too young for sex. In the meantime they teach her how to have safe sex which ensures that she remains a virgin. This is intercrural intercourse – sex between the thighs – in which young women and men must have expertise. When the older women feel that the young sister knows how to perform and how to deal with a man who wants to go beyond the thighs, they give permission for the lovers to have sex. The man pays a small sum of money to the sisters with which they buy a blanket and the remainder is for bread and tea, eaten when they celebrate their sister's sexual maturity. The young woman uses the blanket to sleep with her lover. He comes at night and knocks on the window previously identified for him to ensure that he does not wake up the adults. The young woman takes her blanket and quietly goes out and they both spend the night in a nearby field. They must part company early in the morning whilst it is dark so that no one knows she has been out for the night. But everyone knows that she has reached this sexual stage because as soon as the sisters give permission, the man gets the longest pole he can find, attaches a big white flag on one end and sticks it up by the cattle kraal in his home. People will know it signals his pride.

Whilst the woman is taught how to practise intercrural sex, it is incumbent upon the man, who also gets training from his older brothers not to force himself on the woman. If he does and he breaks the hymen, or impregnates her, he will be charged for 'damages' and will pay a fine in the form of one cow, normally referred to as 'mother's cow', a euphemism for a girl's hymen. If pregnancy occurs there is no argument but if only the hymen has been broken this may need some expertise to detect it. That expertise is available in 'women elders' of the village who can tell that a woman has lost her virginity by simply looking at her eyes or the calf of her legs. If the woman denies the allegation, then an examination settles the issue. Such an action was supported by an annual examination of all unmarried women at the chief's residence. If a woman was found to be without a hymen she is asked to identify the man responsible. He is fined by the chief as well as paying the mother of the girl. If he says he is not responsible then further pressure is put on the woman to say who did it. If she insists that he did it, then the question is why did she not tell her elder sisters when the damage was done if he forced himself on her?

In stage three the man approaches the parents of the woman to ask for her hand in marriage. This is the engagement period. He sends his relatives who negotiate the lobolo (bridewealth). In some cases it can take years before the groom can pay all the lobolo. Sometimes, only part is paid before the wedding. During the engagement the prospective son-in-law is allowed to sleep with his fiancé in the parent's house. He is treated like a celebrity with special food prepared for him. The intercrural intercourse continues.

Stage four starts with the wedding night. Before the wedding the bride-to-be has another lesson about how she should behave in marriage, how and when to have sex with her husband. This time it is full intercourse, not just for pleasure but also for the procreation of children.

Although what I have described relates to South Africa I did discuss these stages with a Nigerian colleague, just to check if the practice went beyond the boundaries of South Africa:

> Oh yes, but you are very soft down there in South Africa. In Nigeria on the first wedding night the in-laws do not go to sleep. They wait for the morning and if the white sheet has no blood on it, the woman is told to take all her belongings and leave. Not only does she lose her husband, but no one in that area would ever marry her.

What became of such practices? Answers may point to Western culture in the guise of Christianity. In Christian teaching, sex before marriage became a mortal sin. Young people's sexual desires and sexual activities were driven underground. That, coupled with an overall rejection of African cultural life and a preference for Western lifestyle put a nail in African custom and practice.

I do not want to give the impression that women's experiences in all these stages were wonderful, and I am certainly not making a case to return to them. Neither am I supporting the double standard morality which force virginity on women but not on men.

Without the humiliation, there is a case for sex education which incorporates intercrural sex. A lot of young people reach a stage in their physical and hormonal development when they want sexual activity. Intercrural sex can offer an outlet and therefore treating sex as part of the complex cultural experience ensures that young women grow up with no 'hang ups' about their own sexuality. It would reduce the number of sexually transmitted diseases.

Although many urban areas have moved away from such sex education, there are pockets in rural areas where it still exists. There is merit in exploring how traditional African sex education can play a part in the fight against AIDS. African sex education, with necessary modification offers clues in thinking about community education and expectations.

Counselling

The seminars stressed the need for sensitivity when dealing with sexual issues. Women reported feeling embarrassed talking about sex-related health issues. If health staff hold hostile attitudes then women will be even more reluctant to use health services. In a training session I attended a Regional AIDS Director stressed that:

- counsellors should listen to the client;
- they should find out the history, cultural beliefs, attitude and knowledge about HIV/AIDS;
- they should not judge the person's sexual behaviour or lack of knowledge. Some men and women have had anal sex. The role of the counsellor is not to bring her attitude about sexual behaviour but to explore with the client how to have safe anal sex;
- they should provide easy to understand information. Many women are frightened that their husbands will infect them. Counselling should offer clients a number of options to take. Some are already infected or have already developed AIDS and will need a lot of physical and emotional support;
- counsellors should have at their fingertips all available services and what supports are available to people with AIDS.

The extent to which women are disempowered and endangered by their subordinate position was brought up in an interview with staff in a surgery. They reported that when a person applies for insurance, the company asks that the person has a medical, including a blood test. The results from the laboratory are sent to the company which sends them back to the doctor who then informs the applicant. Only some of the people who come to this doctor are regular patients:

> It is very hard to break the news when you know people so well. The recent case we have had is really heart breaking. Mrs N is an old patient of ours. She is a very respectable woman, a nursing sister in a clinic. She came for the test because she wanted an educational insurance for her children. When the results came back, she was positive. Her husband drinks and sleeps around with young women. She knows that he is responsible for her infection, but she is frightened of telling him about the results because she knows he will say it is she who has brought the virus into their relationship. She is in a terrible state of tension, and we can't really do anything to help. The doctor has suggested that the next time the husband visits the surgery, he would persuade him to have a general blood check in relation to his drinking and suggest at the same time that he has an HIV test. If he is HIV positive that would open up discussion between him and his wife. The interesting thing is that he has not been to the surgery for the last six months, and yet before all this he used to come

in at least once in two months. I have a very strong suspicion that he knows what is happening. I think he probably had a test himself and knows he is positive but does not want to tell his wife. The whole thing is making their relationship very difficult with this cloud hanging over them and not being able to discuss it and give each other support.

The position in which black women are placed in society remains critical in their overall well-being. The persistent poverty they face and the strategies they employ to combat that poverty pre-dispose them to illnesses. Their health status is further undermined by the violence they face from society and their families.

Violence Against Women

The definition of violence adopted by the World Health Organisation (WHO) is:

> ...any act of gender-based violence that results in, or is likely to result in, physical, sexual, or mental harm or suffering to women, including threats of such acts, coercion or arbitrary deprivation of liberty, whether occurring in public or in private life. This includes, physical, sexual and psychological violence occurring in the family and in the general community, including battering, sexual abuse of children, dowry-related violence, rape, female genital mutilation and other traditional practices harmful to women, non-spousal violence and violence related to exploitation, sexual harassment and intimidation at work, in educational institutions and elsewhere, trafficking in women, forced prostitution and violence perpetrated or condoned by the State (WHO, 1996).

It is important to note that violence against women is a global phenomenon, experienced by women irrespective of their culture, race, or class. Studies conducted in 24 countries on four continents showed that between 20 percent and 50 percent of women were victims of physical abuse by their partners at some stage in their lives and that on average, 50 percent to 60 percent of these abused women are raped by their partners. The perpetrators are almost exclusively men and the greatest risk is from men who are known to the women. In intimate relationships physical abuse is invariably accompanied by severe psychological and verbal abuse (WHO, 1996).

In England, a Training Pack for Domestic Violence in 1994, gave the following national statistics:

- approximately one in ten women have been victims of abuse;
- forty eight percent of murders with a female victim are a result of domestic violence;
- one in five British marriages/partnerships are affected by domestic violence;
- sixty one percent of rapes occur indoors, committed by men known to the victim;
- only one in five of domestic violence incidences are reported to the police. On average, a victim of domestic violence will have been assaulted 35 times before contacting the police;
- forty five percent of female homicide victims are killed by present or former partners.

In South Africa the figures on violence against women are constantly rising. From 1974 to 1995 there was a steady annual increase from 14,815 to 36,888. Assaults went up by 24 percent, murder by 119 percent and rape by 149 percent (National Council of Women of South Africa, 1997). For South African theorists, the increase is explained as an effect of a crisis in masculinity occasioned by a combination of apartheid and capitalism. Two examples conclude this section.

Nomusa's story

> I have had a difficult life. He earned good money, but he only gave me money to buy mealie-meal. He used to say let us buy meat and eat it and not give it to the children. I told him that if my children were not going to eat the meat, neither was I. He would get very angry and I would know that at night when the children were asleep, he would beat me up. I never used to cry because I did not want to upset the kids. I then started making my own money. I used to knock on white people's doors and buy old clothes which I then sold to black people, again by knocking at people's doors. I bought myself a sewing machine and started sewing sheets, bedspreads and curtains. When I made a bit of money he wanted it and if I refused to give it to him, he beat me up. A few days before he fell ill, he threw a carton of milk and it caught the side of my face and the milk went all over me. He was ill for three months and when he died he was totally paralysed. I nursed him to the end. Just before he died, he asked me to forgive him for everything, and I did.

Thandi's story

The story was related by a woman who went to the funeral of Thandi's husband who died suddenly:

> I have never seen anything like it. We were all sitting there and all church men were giving their last respects to this man who they said was the best father and husband. They all said it will be hard for his family to survive without him. You know all the nice things that people say when somebody has died. They sort of made him out to be a saint. Well, Thandi must have had enough. She undid her blouse and knelt in the middle of the floor and said, 'let me show you how good my husband was. He inflicted these bleeding marks on my back last night just before he had the heart attack. If you look closely you will see the old wealds beneath. There was hardly a night when he did not beat me up'. Her back was covered with red bleeding marks where the skin had been cut open. She had never mentioned this to anyone, not even her family.

Nomusa and her husband are a working class couple and Thandi is middle-class. Irrespective of their class, many black women endure violence in their lives. Yet it has not totally disempowered black women, instead it has propelled many forward and in post apartheid South Africa, women are making 'herstory'.

References

Blane, D. (1991), 'Inequality and Social Class' in Scambler, G. (ed), *Sociology as Applied to Medicine*, Bailliere Tindale.

Campbell, R. Coleman, S. and Torkington, N.P.K. (1996), *Street Prostitution in Inner City Liverpool*, Liverpool Hope University College.

Cape Times, 3 July (1997).

Doyle, P. and Muhr, T. (1997), *Seventh Nation HIV Survey of Women Attending Ante-natal Clinics of the Public Health Services*, October/November, Metropolitan Life Ltd.

EUROPAP (1994), *Final Report*, Department of Public Health, Gent, Belgium.

Faugier, J. Hayes, C. and Butterworth, C. (1992), *Drug Using Prostitutes, their Health Care Needs and their Clients*, University of Manchester.

Finchman *et al* (1993), *Department of Health and Population Development: 1991 Health Trends in South Africa*, Pretoria, South Africa.

Gail-Bekker, L. (1998), 'Women and Health Care', *Health Systems Trust Update*, Issue No.31, February, South Africa.

Kelly, K. (1998), *New Directions in Sexual Ethics: Moral Theology and the Challenge of AIDS*, Geoffrey Chapman.

Lund Committee (1996), *Report of the Lund Committee on Child and Family Support*, Department of Health, Pretoria, South Africa.

National Council of Women of South Africa (1997), 'The Rights of Women – Violence/Rape', *Journal of the National Council of Women of South Africa,* vol.65, No.1, January.

Rakgoadi, S. (1997), *Decriminalisation of Sex Work,* sylvester R @ gpg.gov.za.

Sterling, D. (1988), *Black Foremothers,* The Feminist Press: New York.

United Nations (1978), *South African Migrants' Report U.N. Notes and Documents,* Centre against Apartheid.

WHO (1996), *Violence Against Women,* http:www.who.ch/inf/fs/fact128-htlm.

6 Women Making 'Herstory'

Addressing members of the National Council of Women of South Africa at their 1997 conference in Johannesburg, Marlene Bethlehem (1997) stated that all over the world women hold up half the sky insofar as maintaining family life.

In South Africa black women working individually or as groups, have for years struggled not only against gender inequalities but also racial and class oppression. Their struggle has always been related to issues that matter to them, issues that affect their families and most particularly their children. Even before the apartheid regime women fought against discriminatory laws.

In 1913, the year of the Land Act which formally gave white people 87 percent of land and black people 13 percent, saw the formation of the Bantu Women's League, the first political organisation for black women in South Africa. The League laid the foundation for the African National Congress (ANC) Women's League which was later to play a crucial role in the fight against Pass Laws. Under apartheid women continued the fight.

In 1954 the Federation of South African Women was formed with the aim of securing freedom for all as well as an improvement in the quality of women's life. To this end this organisation with others such as the ANC Women's League, challenged all racist laws which included the Natives Land Act, the Natives Resettlement Bill and the Bantu Education Bill. In consequence Bethlehem points out that women were disproportionately active in housing struggles, because in practice they were the ones who established homes and took care of the children. In this sense women's political action was linked to their identities as mothers and caregivers. This pattern continued in the 1980s, with women playing a strong role in anti-detention campaigns, struggles over rent and housing and support for political prisoners.

The issues that women addressed in the past remain pertinent today: i.e. the education of children, housing and employment. To this list we add violence against women and children and in particular, rape. This is not to say that in the past rape was unheard of, but rather to emphasise the high incidence among young children. The rise in social and political problems is matched by the rise in the number of women's organisations. As the list below shows, each of the nine provinces has a number of active women's groups.

Table 6.1 Women's organisations in the nine provinces

Province	Number of women's organisations
Eastern Cape	118
Eastern Transvaal	26
Free State	54
Gauteng	279
KwaZulu-Natal	211
North West	39
Northern Cape	31
Northern Province	50
Western Cape	148

Source: Barnard (1995).

It is safe to assume that the above figures are an underestimate since many small organisations, particularly in rural areas, would not have known about the compilation of this data and would therefore not be included. It is equally safe to assume that the majority of the organisations will be composed of black women. This is because there are more black people than white people in South Africa and also because the social and political issues which gave rise to these organisations affected black women more than white women.

Although only 169 of these organisations are health specific, with 178 falling under the related category of welfare, social and community services, a broader definition of health would suggest that even those organisations which are not overtly related to health have a positive impact on the health of the community.

While it is not possible to profile each organisation to demonstrate this fact some of the women's organisations described in this chapter are illustrative. The selection of these organisations was not random. They are based in areas where fieldwork for this research was undertaken or had representatives who were available for interview. Thus opportunism featured in the sampling. Although they have a specific health brief, their overall work has positive influences on the general health of communities in which they are based. Some have a long history, others are relatively new, building on the work of earlier organisations as well as addressing new problems. In this chapter I consider the work of organisations in urban and rural areas sharing two characteristics – their concern for the health and welfare of families and their voluntary bases. I also draw attention to the ideas and approaches to problem solving which women bring into their work. It is this which has earned this chapter the title of 'Women Making Herstory'.

Women's Organisations in Urban Areas

In this section we shall look at four organisations - the National Council of African Women (NCAW), Ikageng, Women's Health and Empowerment Programme, which is part of the National Progressive Primary Health Care Network (NPPHCN), and the Women's Voice of Orange Farm.

National Council of African Women (NCAW)

The origin of this organisation lies in the struggle for leadership by black men over black women in meetings where issues of land were discussed on 16 December 1937. Women were annoyed at having to waste time over leadership instead of tackling more fundamental and far-reaching issues affecting the country and society as a whole. They requested the Chairman to allow them to hold their own meeting. The Chairman agreed and NCAW emerged with Charlotte Maxeke as the Chairperson. Since then some 20,000 branches were formed in different regions. The activities of NCAW are wide ranging. There is concern about the environment. Members of NCAW raise awareness about environmental care and encourage people to participate in the re-cycling of paper, tins and glass. They organise the planting of trees in their areas. Children are drawn into this activity not only because they have important roles in their communities but also to develop a sense of ownership which will promote their interest in nurturing the young trees.

Health

Members are also active in the field of health. They are involved at two levels – assisting in the provision of health services and developing preventative health provision. In the past they have assisted in the building of clinics when the Nationalist government was least concerned about this service for black people. Preventative health takes the form of creating vegetable gardens. Members encourage women to have vegetable gardens to provide fresh food for their families. There are, however, two initiatives through which NCAW has contributed in making Herstory – Learn and Earn project in prisons and Education.

Learn and Earn Project in Prisons

Members of the organisation are working closely with prison officials to define the role of prisons. If they are cast as corrective institutions, people should acquire skills useful to themselves, their families and the community at large. They suggested an introduction of the Learn and Earn project to enable inmates to acquire skills such as carpentry, plumbing, sewing for example. If these skills do earn money this can be kept in a trust and some of it be given to ex-prisoners. The trust, formed by different women's organisations, is already in existence. Earnings from prisoners augment it. The creation of the trust does not condone the crimes committed. The bottom line is that many of the women associated with the trust are mothers of prisoners, so the women are especially keen to find ways of ensuring that their children do not return to prison. Acquiring skills and a sense of self-worth are the compelling aims of the Learn and Earn project. For South Africa this is a radical approach which, if implemented widely, would revolutionise the prison service nationally.

Education

Historically NCAW has always had a particular interest in education especially that of young girls who were under-represented in the education system. Thus, interest in education has grown as younger women join the Council. Most branches now concentrate on providing financial support to girls and young women in primary, high school and universities. In the

Gauteng province a new need in relation to university students has arisen which has shifted the focus to accommodation.

The concern is on the health and safety of students who are not able to have accommodation in halls either because these are full or they cannot afford the fees. Most of these students find themselves paying high rent in shacks without running water or electricity. They use candles or paraffin lamps for study and use paraffin primus stoves for cooking. They use unhygienic toilets and have no privacy, particularly those who share a room with other family members. These students have little access to libraries in the evenings as it is unsafe to walk at night. Thus, it is not only the education of these students which suffers but their health is also compromised. The problem is more acute in the university of the North. NCAW has negotiated with Home Affairs officials in the area and has been given land to build residential accommodation for the students with library facilities. Members want to incorporate child-care facilities to ensure that the facilities are used by the students and the community. The organisation is currently in the process of finding funding. The students will pay affordable rent which will be used to set up similar services in other provinces.

The Learn and Earn and the student accommodation projects share a common outcome – a reduction in crime committed by young people. In the first project the aim is not only to create self-esteem and self-worth through acquiring skills but is also to provide ex-prisoners with financial support when they leave prison. Without that support some people may be drawn into re-offending in order to survive. The existing penal system is therefore ineffective in reducing crime. The way forward lies in developing a system within which offenders are offered an opportunity to re-gain their confidence, self-worth and self-esteem and have the material means to re-integrate into their communities as responsible citizens. Women are leading in this development and when the Learn and Earn project is established nationally, this will be a landmark in South Africa's judiciary system.

The student accommodation project reduces the chances of young people dropping out of higher education within which their potential to contribute to the development of their country is maximised. But of equal importance is the reduced opportunity to drift into crime as a result of frustration, loss of confidence and self-worth when young people are forced by circumstances to drop out of the education system.

IKAGENG (build yourself)

This organisation was established in 1965 by Marjory Nomsa Mhlala, a woman who was sought in a dream to bring women together to develop the black community. Although the idea first took root at Themba, one of the townships in Gauteng, it soon spread with a total of 72 branches in the country. The Diepkloof branch which I visited was started on 15 March 1973 and had 15 members. Today there are 200 members and the branch is the most active in the Soweto region. The ex-chair, who held the chair for 24 years, informed me that during the apartheid years women were frightened to do community work openly because such activities were wilfully interpreted as political resistance by the government.

Ikageng is the only black women's organisation in which members wear a uniform:

> Before I joined Ikageng I had been exposed to other women's organisations. I found them too superior and class conscious. I remember one in particular where members were criticising the quality of teaspoons as they drank tea provided by a member who was hosting the meeting. Our Organisation takes women from all walks of life - housewives, domestic workers, professionals as well as people who have never been to school, whether or not they have quality teaspoons. As women we are equal and we have equal worth in the work we do for our community. The uniform is a symbol of that equality (Ex Chair, 1997).

The ex-chair stressed that human dignity and community development which the organisation seeks to foster must be evident within the membership. Those who cannot afford to buy expensive clothes for conferences/meetings must not be made to feel lesser or inferior as such feelings are divisive and can undermine collective community work.

The constitution of the organisation focuses on the factors which promote family life e.g. alcohol is seen as the destroyer of families and is not served in Ikageng meetings and conferences. Women learn together about managing their families. In order to extend knowledge which promotes family life the organisation has affiliated to other organisations. The Diepkloof branch extended the constitution by adding a clause which emphasises care for the destitute of all ages. But to do this work the group needed money, so how did they manage?:

We followed our motto which says, 'you women are the light of the world and by hope and faith you shall prosper'. So we did not start by asking people for money. We started from our pockets. We all had small tins in which we put small change from our shopping and to that we added R5 a month. We held cake sales and sold lunches at the time when a plate of food was selling for R3. When the project was up and running we then invited people to come and see what we were doing and advertised ourselves and our food. We invited trusts and business people as well as community groups and individuals. Those who can afford it adopted the whole or part of the project. If you start asking for money before you start a project, you are cheating. It is like asking for a lift while standing still. You have to walk so that people from whom you are asking for a lift can see that you are making an effort (Ex Chair, 1997).

Ikageng enacts this philosophy in the development of many projects.

Nutrition

For years the members have provided money to buy food for children whose families are not able to provide and for those who have no families. As the project expanded they invited companies and trusts to see the project meeting an identified need. Some made a one off contribution and others e.g. McLeans Trust 'adopted' the feeding bill of the project.

Health

In health provision women adopted a similar approach. In 1977 when Kliptown was flooded, its residents were moved to Mzimhlophe – a transit camp formerly used as a hostel. Inkageng women supplied them with food and clothing until they could return to their homes and recover some of their lives. In the meantime it was discovered that children had a variety of diseases – sore eyes, ringworm, scabies and diarrhoea. The clinic was too far away and parents did not have money for transport. Inkageng explored with residents the kinds of help they could give. A clinic for the area was identified as a priority. That they had neither money nor building skills did not stop them. Using the bricks of offices burnt down in the 1976 Children's Uprising, women built a clinic. The invited companies noted that the walls were not straight and were potentially dangerous. Soon after these visits help came in the form of skilled builders from construction companies and money from trusts which 'adopted' nurse's salaries and bills for medicine. The clinic continued to function until 1993 when the hostel riots between members of the ANC and Inkatha made it a no-go area.

Inkageng members are not content in simply providing a service. They also engage in research in order to have evidence on which to base the information and the advice they give to their communities. One such research was on the effects of Depo Provera, a contraceptive widely used in South Africa.

The current thinking at the time was that the Nationalist government was encouraging the use of Depo Provera in order to limit the black population. Not only would the drug reduce the numbers of children born but it would also reduce the number of women as many would die of cancer which came to be associated with this contraceptive. From the study conducted in 1985, Inkageng women concluded that:

> Depo does not cause cancer because women who had not used the drug also had cancer. It did not cause infertility but only delayed ovulation in some women. Others got pregnant soon after coming off the drug. If used after giving birth Depo helps the uterus to go back to its original position quickly. We also found out that there is not enough education on contraceptives in general. Some women believed that they only had to take the pill when they have sex, they do not know that the pill must be in their blood in order to prevent ovulation (Ex Chair, 1997).

These findings enabled members of Ikangeng to identify gaps in people's knowledge about contraceptives in general and more specifically about Depo Provera using evidence-based knowledge. The findings of the research formed part of the material disseminated in health workshops attended by women.

Fostering

Ikageng has a unique and healthy approach to fostering. If a mother falls ill after delivery and there is no one in the family to look after the baby, social workers find a foster home. As this process takes a long time Ikageng finds someone to look after the baby. That person is usually a member of the organisation who is not in paid employment. The group provides the same service for older children.

In the course of this research an appeal came from one family for help in the fostering of children. Their mother died of cancer leaving six children with their aunt. Unable to meet the bills, the aunt appealed to the group for food and the payment of electricity and council rates. At the meeting of the group which I attended, a member reported that the aunt was now terminally ill and the children had no one to look after them. The women agreed that they would find someone to look after the children until a relative willing to look after them was found or social workers were able to find a suitable placement for them.

In fostering, particularly that which involves children rather than babies, the group emphasises the importance of not disrupting children's lives further by moving them from their home at a time when they are distressed and bereaved. Thus, instead of moving the children, the foster mother moves into their home until a more permanent placement is arranged. This is in stark contrast with Western-based fostering practices where children are not only moved from their homes but also out of all that is familiar to them. Some social workers accept that this is detrimental to the wellbeing of children:

> I actually think that we need to have community parents so that kids are not moved from all that they know. When we move them we sometimes leave their clothes and toys behind – everything that is comfortable to them. We move them out of their home and community into a different class and sometimes race (Placement Manager, Liverpool, 1999).

The Ikageng women are leading the way in providing sensitive fostering which will have long-term positive effects on the well-being of fostered children.

Community Education

Central to the ethos of Ikageng is the belief that people must do things for themselves. Support and assistance must come to expand rather than to initiate an activity. But the women are also aware that for that to happen people need education, not just classroom education but experiential knowledge about their society, and that includes the roles of central and local government, the constitution, the resources available to communities and knowledge of, for example, human rights. Ikageng arranges meetings and conferences as crucial means of disseminating information to the wider public.

An event I attended was a symposium to introduce the Gauteng Consumer Affairs Department to the Soweto community. The aim was to educate people about what they can do to minimise and resolve consumer problems. The women used drama to highlight some of the problems faced by consumers as well as offering advice such as, reading the small print before signing any agreement, budgeting carefully before buying anything and avoiding using 'plastic cards' unless you know you can cope with payments.

The drama illustrated a variety of problems arising from real life situations - furniture shops refusing to honour guarantees, the long distance of consumer offices from where people live and the inaccessibility of offices for people using wheelchairs.

At the symposium the concept of consumerism was given a broad definition which focused not only on bought goods but also on the role of government in relation to the constitution. The government has already met one obligation, the establishment of a consumer court. But is it a fair court? Is it fair, for example, to tell people to read the small print before signing any contract in a country with high illiteracy rate? Does it make sense to encourage people in wheelchairs to take their cases to the consumer court if there is no access for them? Such services need government intervention if the equality espoused in the constitution is to be a reality for many people in South Africa. Ultimately it is the responsibility of the government to provide education to ensure that people are literate. In the interim giving information other than in the form of the written word is an invitation to local creativity.

Another problem addressed in the symposium highlighted the operation of the new eviction law. The law states that if the worker has been issued with an eviction order then the government will assist in the resettlement of that person. Where no eviction order is in evidence then no government help will be given. Some farmers take advantage of this law, knowingly or not. When they retire they move out of the farm into town flats. They tell their farm workers to move out of the farm and if they do not, because they have no where to go, they dismantle their homes without giving them an eviction order. They claim that they do not know anything about the eviction law and they do not know where to go for information. These are the perverse practices to which the government must attend if equality and human dignity espoused in the constitution is to become a reality.

The symposium was attended by senior staff from the Consumer Affairs Department who had first hand information from the workshops in which a number of suggestions were made. It was suggested that there must be consumer offices in Soweto so that people do not have to travel long distances and spend a lot of money taking their complaints to town. Consumer offices must be located in accessible premises where people pay for services such as rates, electricity and rent. Consumer forums must be established in different parts of the township which could operate as advice and monitoring centres. It was recognised that communities must take responsibility for their own education with volunteers from those who have knowledge of how the system works, and those who will disseminate that information to others. As the women stressed, 'we must educate one another'. The Ikageng women see community education as crucial in enabling people to become active citizens and to use the constitution effectively. Through the constitution the government has declared its commitment to equality and the upholding of human rights, but it is the people who must make the constitution work and they can only do this if they are informed. This point was stressed by a speaker at the symposium:

> The government has given us the constitution, but if we sit and wait for the government to do things for us we are missing the point. The Constitution empowers us to do things for ourselves. We must encourage the formation of social solidarity groups which will adhere to humane values which see my power as your power, my knowledge as your knowledge. Unless we are prepared to organise along these lines, the constitution will remain a theoretical pronouncement (Speaker, 1997).

Women's Health and Empowerment Programme (WHEP)

WHEP is part of the National Progressive Primary Health Care Network (NPPHCN). The network started in 1987 and its history is rooted in the politics of the apartheid regime. Before 1976 ninety five percent of doctors working in the townships were white. With the uprisings of 1976 many of these doctors closed their practices in the townships. This created a crisis as people were left without primary care. To address the problem courses were arranged for nurses to enable them to diagnose and treat minor ailments in clinics. However, this shifted people's perception of primary health care, they saw it as being treated by a nurse rather than a doctor. The network had its origins in correcting this misconception. A group of professionals from the anti-apartheid movement came together to form the network which aimed to promote a more inclusive concept of primary health care. To achieve this task the network adopted the concept used at the Conference at Alma Ata in 1978 which stated that a progressive health care approach is about challenging the society to address the socio-economic causes of poor health and making provision for basic health needs in a way that encourages community empowerment. It is about providing a comprehensive quality health care system which includes promotive, preventive, curative, rehabilitative and palliative services in a way that demands commitment and accountability from health workers. It is about prioritising disadvantaged groups to ensure that health care is accessible, equitable and affordable to all. A progressive health care approach must recognise the importance of integrated service provision from primary to tertiary levels of care within a coherent health care system and must promote interdisciplinary, multi-professional and intersectoral collaborative teamwork for development.

The mission of the NPPHCN is to promote primary health care in the following ways:

- advocating (influencing, mobilising, and lobbying) for a national primary health care policy and its implementation;
- transferring appropriate skills to community based organisations;
- bringing together members to share information, skills and experiences;
- providing practical support to members (NPPHCN leaflet).

The network has gone through a number of phases. The first phase was between 1987 and 1992 when black people were discriminated against in the distribution of resources and in treatment. Many members of the network took a political stand and fought against the discriminatory practices. The second phase was from 1992 when restrictions were removed from the African National Congress. This brought about a change in attitude. Prior to this, political activists who were employed by the government were seen as part of the oppressive system. After 1992 there was a move to enter employment in government offices to find out what was happening in preparation for the new government. This coincided with the perhaps self-seeking Nationalist Party's strategy of opening doors to black people in certain areas of employment. This was the period of transition during which the network, together with other political organisations, helped in the formulation of a health policy for the new South Africa.

The third phase started in 1994 with the emergence of the ANC government when the organisation became a focus for debate. Now that the apartheid regime has gone, was it still necessary to have the network? The consensus was that NPPHCN should continue to operate as a watchdog for the people. This was seen as a crucial role in the health service:

> We support and work closely with the new government. Even now we are involved in the drafting of the documents for the National Health Act which will be ready before the end of this year. But we are equally critical of some of the policies. We stand for people. People should be empowered so that they participate fully and effectively in health and all other areas which affect their lives (WHEP Co-ordinator, 1997).

This is not an easy task considering the size of the population in relation to trained doctors and nurses. It is for this reason that the network introduced the concept of community health workers.

The introduction of community health workers arose from the conviction that health must be rooted in people's daily experiences. The training of local people in basic health care would have two functions: involve people in their own health and empower them. In the government's draft of its National Health Service, there was a paragraph on the role of community health workers, but in the final document, this was removed even though there were already some trained community health workers. In some areas they were paid and in others they were working as volunteers. This unequal treatment along with their invisibility at a national level has created confusion, resentment and has weakened some community worker's commitment. The co-ordinator for WHEP is confident, however, that the government will reconsider when it sees the value of community health care workers whose role combines curative, promotive and preventative health care.

NPPHCN members were working with the government in drafting the 12th Bill which, it was hoped, would emerge as the National Health Act before the end of 1997. Reference to and promotion of health care workers in the Act would be a great asset to many communities, especially those in remote rural areas with poor health facilities.

The success of NPPHCN to achieve its objectives will be determined by resources in the form of funding and the workforce, both of which have been weakened since the establishment of the new government.

Many of the senior staff involved in formulating health policy during the period of transition were subsequently offered jobs by the government thus reducing the number of experienced workers for the network. Some have become Members of Parliament, provincial premiers and directors in the health service. Another difficulty has been posed by funders who have been providing financial support during the apartheid regime. Some of them have now stopped funding NGOs and are giving their money directly to the government. This money has not always found its way to where it is needed and as a result, good work has been disrupted at community level. One example is provided by USNID. This had been funding work on AIDS and switched its funding to the government. The network lost 58 AIDS field workers who were immersed in community education at grass root level and running workshops in various parts of the country. The government's approach to combating AIDS created the R14 million scandal when the money was given to a producer to educate the public through drama in the theatre. Even if this was an effective way of disseminating information on AIDS, which many South Africans say it was not, how many people access the theatre in urban areas never mind in rural ones? These difficulties, however, have not stopped the work of the network which has divided itself into four main national wings, one of which is the Women's Health and Empowerment Programme.

Like all the other national wings of the network, WHEP works in all provinces enabling people to do things for themselves. As part of the empowerment process, the development of leadership is fostered to make sure that things do not come to a standstill when the facilitator leaves the area. The organisation relies heavily on community-based voluntary work for community education. The overarching aim is to establish women's groups in all provinces which will advance the education of women.

Nutrition

As nutrition for children from birth to school age is so important WHEP is working with the government on its breastfeeding campaign. The government wants to target clinics and maternity hospitals to encourage women to breastfeed their infants. WHEP believes that the campaign must be community-based, starting with women before they even become pregnant so that by the time they deliver, they understand the advantages of breastfeeding. The message must not only come from facilitators but be reinforced by local people who have had children and credibly talk from experience. Experience shows that when a message comes from the community to the community it carries more weight than when it comes from health professionals who are not part of that community. It should not be difficult, argues the WHEP national co-ordinator, to encourage breastfeeding.

Some women have been brainwashed to believe that bottle-feeding with formulae milk is the best, others, however, are caught up in beliefs and myths which need to be tackled. There is a belief that colostrum, the clear fluid which the breast produces during the few days after delivery, is dangerous for the baby. So, many women do not breastfeed until the breasts start producing milk. In reality, colostrum is the most needed nutrient because it is rich not only in vitamins and other nutritional elements but also in anti-bodies. Some women believe that having sexual intercourse whilst breastfeeding harms the baby. This belief renders bottle feeding an attractive option. WHEP wants to understand the influence of such beliefs to ensure that women are not distracted from breastfeeding their babies. Their overall aim is to nurture safe and healthy motherhood.

In schools WHEP is promoting the feeding scheme for primary school children started by the government in 1996. It argues that in providing the food, local women's organisations must be involved not only for socio-economic empowerment reasons but also because it makes sense for schools. When big companies provide food for schools they do not serve it to the children. They deliver it and the teachers serve it or find volunteer women to do the job. This is exploitative to the women and is not the most appropriate way of using teacher's time. If the contract was given to women's organisations, women would not only provide the food, but would also serve it to the children.

Women's Reproductive Rights

WHEP is heavily involved in women's reproductive rights. A pre-occupying theme has been the legalisation of abortion in South Africa. Workshops were held in different parts of the country to explain to women what the Bill means and why the government wants to legalise abortion i.e. to limit the number of deaths from back street abortions. As the co-ordinator observes, the question is not whether women should have abortions:

> They have already made their choice. They go to the back streets. Nothing new is being introduced here. The government is looking at the situation from a public health point of view (WHEP Co-ordinator, 1997).

A National Health survey conducted by Hirschwitz and Orkin (1995) showed that less that 30 percent favoured legal abortion. Africans at 28 percent were the least in favour compared to 47 percent Europeans who favoured the Bill. Since the country is divided on whether or not abortion should be legalised, would a referendum help?:

> Not really if our concern is about the danger of street abortion to women. Half of the women who said abortion should not be legalised had had street abortions themselves. Just because people have had abortions this does not mean that they will say it is a good thing and endorse it' (WHEP Co-ordinator, 1997).

There are obviously differences between expressed preferences and what people do and this is evidenced in the abortion debate.

The role of WHEP is not to campaign for abortion but to explain to women what the legislation is about and to advise women about contraception to avoid pregnancy in the first instance. If they still want to terminate a pregnancy, they need to know that there are safer alternatives to back street abortion.

The three organisations discussed have a number of common factors. They were set up because of concerns about matters that affect women. They were established to support and empower women in their efforts to maintain their families in a society that discriminated against them because they were women, black and economically powerless. These organisations worked and continue to work for and on behalf of women. They have developed branches in different parts of the country which focus on specific needs of their localities but within the guidelines of the mother organisation.

The next group, Women's Voice of Orange Farm, has a slightly different origin in that it was set up by women to attend to their day-to-day needs. Members must be involved in project work and that ensures that the organisation is not a 'talking shop' but a hands-on reality. The group is seeking economic stability to ensure that its activities continue. To do this, members are engaged in economic activities that were once the preserve of men.

Women's Voice of Orange Farm

This is a consortium of 12 groups of women. Each group selects two women who represent it in the Executive Committee. Since 1989 the Committee has been illegally squatting in the Government Administrative Offices in Orange Farm. The Chair said:

> We have been here since 1989. We use their phones, their electricity, their fax and their rooms. They phone me now and again to tell me that we must vacate their premises. I tell them, if you trust yourself come and remove me or send someone you trust to remove me. We have told them that all they need to do to get rid of us is to give us a site where we can build our own centre (Chair).

These were not empty challenges from a formidable woman in stature, confidence, knowledge and political acumen. The women were eventually given a site where they will build their community centre. Although still involved in long established, gender specific roles, these women are crossing boundaries and adopting new working roles.

The Environment and Agricultural Project

The impetus for this project was the ownership of land by the women. They have a farm beyond the Orange Farm settlement. The farm was one of the many expropriated by the previous government. The chair applied for the farm and it was given to her for R720 rent a month. The ANC government has stipulated that this land must be used for agricultural purposes. In the past few years the chair has lived in the house and used the rooms for different women's projects including sewing classes. Preparations are now on the way to start farming. Within this project women will form themselves into groups. Each member of the group will have five hectares on which to grow vegetables for commercial purposes as well as subsistence. The women will have a ready-made market in crèches that are already co-ordinated by women who will be members of the project. But to ensure a sustainable, secure and long-term market, the women are already negotiating with the government to give them a contract to supply schools with fresh vegetables. The amount of land available is so huge that the intention is to use some of it for pastoral farming. There will be the usual rearing of cattle, but in addition women will be free to try their hand in other areas such as poultry and pig farming for example.

The work of women in this field has attracted a lot of interest. Murray and Roberts, the biggest construction company in South Africa, has donated R1.5 million to purchase land on which to build an agricultural college. With this money the women have already bought land adjacent to the farm they already own. Israel, through Begurion University of Negev has donated R5 million to the project and they will provide agricultural experts on irrigation, soil testing and the maximisation of the produce with environmental safety in mind. They will also provide lecturers until such time that indigenous people are trained to take on those jobs. Financial support has also come from the Royal Netherlands through a woman who came to South Africa to oversee the elections in 1994. She stayed on and got involved with projects and has since linked the farming project with funders in Holland. Under the present government's New Farmer Settlement Scheme, the women now qualify for a subsidy, an initial sum of R25,000 per person. The chair is exuberant:

> I have always wanted land for women. Just to have it was my goal in life. We shall have space to build a farmers' resource centre for every type of equipment that the groups will need (Chair, 1997).

The college will operate on a fee-paying basis for non-members. Members will probably not pay or pay a nominal fee. Other women who cannot afford to pay will be considered for training. The college will be open to all. The two most exciting things about this Environment and Agricultural project are that the college will be built by women, and the women will be taught to employ organic methods in the production of food.

The drive for the environment side of the project is as strong as the business side. Women are keen to create parks for the townships and they are going to encourage tree planting using schemes that will motivate the communities to be involved in this. People will learn about how and when to water their plants to ensure that water is not wasted. Women are also aware that recycling is preserving nature's resources.

Women in Business

Whilst some women remain involved in small-scale businesses such as street hawking, owning 'spaza shops', candle-making and sewing, others are succeeding in areas which challenge the patriarchal officialdom which still believes that certain jobs can only be done by men.

The Construction Industry

When the programme of building toilets in Orange Farm was introduced, the tender for the making of bricks and building the toilets was given to men, even though women had submitted tenders. Women did not challenge this, instead they asked for the brick making to be sub-contracted to them. When the Council checked the quality of bricks made, they found that almost all the bricks made by men failed the checks, but those made by women passed. It transpired that men were helping themselves to the cement which meant that their bricks were mainly made of sand and that is why they crumbled when tested.

The pattern in the quality of the bricks was so persistent that eventually the Council withdrew the contract from some men, for both brick making and toilet building, and gave it to women contractors. Other women who are not contractors continue to make bricks as a co-operative and they supply women contractors whilst others continue to sub-contract to men. A factor which has strengthened the position of women in this area is the link made with educational institutions.

The Role of Educational Institutions in the Empowerment of Women

One of the strategies adopted by the Women's Voice of Orange Farm has been the formation of a partnership with institutions of education. One of these institutions is Technikon Witwaterand. The major link is the head of the Planning Department. In the past black students have had difficulty finding opportunities for field work in their architectural and planning studies. Now the link with the women in Orange Farm has given them new opportunities:

> It is a healthy partnership from which we all benefit. The black students have their placement with us and through that they get their qualification. When they are with us they train us so that we become competent when we take on building work (Committee member, 1997).

In fact the partnership goes beyond this initial contact. When these students qualify they will have links with communities that will provide them with employment opportunities. Their placement teaches them not only about bricks and mortar but also about how they should work with communities in the process of growing. For the women the benefits include acquiring building skills and being part of projects for which they are paid. A potential project is the renovation of Stretford Station in Orange Farm. The Council has given this job to Technikon Witwaterand. The Technikon hopes to employ the women to do the work under the existing partnership with the students. The institution will take responsibility to ensure that the work is done to the highest standard. The Technikon is so confident that the women are capable of this standard that they have suggested that the women should also renovate its own buildings and build their own college of agriculture:

> The students have already drawn the plans for our college. The women are going to make the bricks and do the building under the guidance of the Technikon and its students on placement. We are all very excited about this project (Committee member, 1997).

Another big building programme for the women has been offered by the residents of Orange Farm who still live in shacks. The procedure is for residents of any area to apply for funding from the RDP. The amount for each house is R15,000. In Orange Farm men have been given the tender to build these houses.

On my first visit to Orange Farm I was able to see a finished product of one room measuring about nine square metres. Inside was a double bed which almost occupied the whole room. There was just enough space for a dressing table. On one side was a primus stove on which the owner had just cooked lunch. On the other side he kept his pans and a bucket of water. He was sitting on the bed eating his lunch when I asked if I could see his house. Outside, attached to the house was what I thought was a carport with a concrete floor. The space was almost as big as the room. I was informed that this was not a carport but an area in which the owner may wish to build another room in the future. At the end of this space was a sink and a toilet, neither of which were functioning. Outside was a communal water tap and people came from afar to use it. I asked the owner what he thought of his new home:

> Well it is not ideal but it is better than being in a shack. The problem is that it is too small and only one room. We have two children and there is no room here so I can't bring them and my wife until I have found some way of enclosing the space outside for another room.

Some people had already enclosed the area using the same materials they had used in building their shacks. The people who wanted to move out of the shacks wanted four-roomed houses with the R15,000 and the Women's Voice of Orange Farm were promising them that. But is this feasible?:

> Yes it is. You see all that money will go to buying material. On this one we are working with the students from Potchefstroom University. The students who are on placement with us have already done the plans. That means we do not have to pay for architects. When we build toilets in this area we are going to teach women there how to make bricks and how to build, so by the time we come to build their houses they will be making the bricks and taking part in building their own homes. The University will supervise and monitor the building process. The students will work with the women training them in the skills of house building. At the end of the day everyone has had the reward. The students get the satisfaction of being involved in the development of the communities for which they get their academic credits towards their degrees. The women? Well the rewards here are at different levels. There are the women who will have their houses on the land they own for the first time. That is a big incentive to be involved. For those who build these houses for the residents there is a gain in the form of understanding why there is so little money available and the opportunity to be imaginative in using that little money to develop their communities. You see, unlike men, women are prepared to do this on a voluntary basis if there is no money to pay for their labour (Chair, 1997).

Although the basic building will be the norm for the R15,000 there is no reason why those families who can afford can't put in extra money to have more than the basic house:

We anticipate that the houses here will all be different, reflecting the level of ability of individual families to contribute towards their own homes. Already there are employers who have offered financial assistance to their workers. We are also looking out for sponsorships because we want to do a good job. But whether or not we get that sponsorship, with the R15,000 we are going to build decent four roomed houses for our communities (Committee member, 1997).

The involvement of women in building projects suggests that in future women have the potential to play an important role in the construction industry. If that happens we may begin to see more imaginative planning and house designing since the people who spend most of their time in the house will be involved in those processes.

Refuse Collection from the Townships

When the township councils terminated existing contracts with refuse collecting services, the women put in a tender for a new contract. They were confident of wining the contract because of the approach they wanted to employ. They were going to be cheap because they were not going to use expensive trucks for collecting refuse. They were going to involve every member of the community. People were going to be encouraged to use whatever means they had to bring refuse to a designated centre – buckets, wheelbarrows and vans, and they would be paid for every kilo of rubbish brought to the Centre.

In collecting refuse women also wanted to implement the environmental principles of preserving nature's resources. There would be special days for specific forms of rubbish. There would be a day for kitchen refuse such as leftover food and a day for garden rubbish. These products would find their way to the women's agricultural farm to be used as organic fertiliser instead of chemicals, with positive implications for the quality of the vegetables produced as well as the environment. There would be 'dedicated' days for paper, glass and tins. The women wanted to make links with recycling firms:

> There will be enough incentive for people to be involved in cleaning their own areas. First of all people will have pride in knowing that they have been personally involved in cleaning up the area. They will be concerned if other people make it dirty and their disapproval will be made in no

unclear terms. But also people will know that they will get paid for removing the rubbish. Whilst the project is running no one can say there is no work. Even though the amount of money will be limited, still there will be a chance to earn something instead of just sitting at home (Committee member, 1997).

If the women get the tender it will be the most imaginative method of cleaning the townships. But even if they do not get the tender, such originality, imagination and pragmatism cannot be overlooked indefinitely.

Masakhane Campaign

In the past one of the ways of protesting against the apartheid system in the provision of services had been to withhold payments for council services. The consequence is that many people have become accustomed to non-payment for services and persist in not paying their bills under the post-apartheid government. The result is that councils are starved of funds and are unable to provide the services. To resolve this problem, the government launched a campaign called Masakhane (let us build each other) aiming to encourage people to pay their rates. As part of this campaign the Southern Metropolitan Substructure put out a tender for organisations to get a contract to deliver monthly statements on services to all families who were not paying their rents. The Women's Voice of Orange Farm planned to take part in this venture. The women intended to undertake some action research. They knew that there were a lot of reasons why people did not pay their bills in addition to habit. The women believed that many people would be prepared to pay if they were given usable information including a breakdown of the amounts they pay for specific services. Some people did not pay because they were unemployed. Others could not decipher the forms because of poor literacy. Part of the problem was poor communication skills:

> One of the problems is that nobody actually sits down and addresses service delivery issues with individual families. People get statements about rates but they do not understand the information on these statements. Some people look at the registration number and think it is the amount of money they have to pay and give up the thought of paying. Literacy classes are needed to enable people to access information not only on rates but all services and issues that affect their lives locally,

nationally and internationally. We believe that when people do not understand they become frustrated and then they start to fight and the cause is lost. If people understand what they are paying for, then you will find that many will pay. But we are not just going to concentrate on payment, we are going to write everything down that people tell us about their problems and we are going to call counsellors and all relevant people to discuss all issues that will arise from this work and try and find solutions collectively (Committee member, 1997).

The information collected will be used to make a persuasive case with government departments for jobs for the unemployed.

Health and Welfare Forum

This is a general group in which the Women's Voice of Orange Farm is represented. The forum brings together people with health interests such as doctors, social workers, nurses, teachers, counsellors and representatives from community groups. The group meets once a month to review health related matters. It is to this group that the women primary health care workers are linked.

Primary health care workers are women drawn from the community and trained for three months by the St John's ambulance in conjunction with Technikon South Africa which issues certificates for successful participants. The women then undertake a further three-month course which qualifies them as district health care workers. After this course they are competent to deal with specific health needs such as minor burns, sprains and bedsores. They can check blood pressure and they advise family members what to do if someone has an epileptic fit. They demonstrate re-hydration procedures in order to enable parents to treat their own babies when they have vomiting and diarrhoea. They also tell parents to look out for indicators of dehydration such as sunken eyes and loose skin. The emphasis is on starting treatment before these signs manifest themselves. They inform mothers about the signs and symptoms of child abuse. They advise on how mothers should make themselves accessible to their children so that they will not be secretive when they get abused. They also advise children not to accept gifts or talk to strangers in potentially dangerous areas. Serious heath problems are always referred to clinics, surgeries, and hospitals. All activities are referred to the Health and Welfare Forum.

Women working as midwives are untrained. They are drawn from the 'Wise Women of the Village' whose skills in childbirth have been passed from generation to generation. In the past they have been dismissed by Western-endorsed midwifery as ignorant and illiterate. Now their methods are being re-examined and are found to have enormous merit in enabling women to have more natural childbirth. Some training is needed to extend the skills of these workers to identify problems in all stages of pregnancy and childbirth and refer the women to the appropriate agencies.

All health community workers work on a voluntary basis. There is dawning recognition of their importance by the government and some hope that they may ultimately actually be paid, with the potential for a credible community based service to grow and serve South Africa.

Siyaphambili (we go Forward) Early Learning Project

A pre-occupying concern for the women in Orange Farm is the welfare of children, for their health and their safety. Many children live in homes where they are either left to fend for themselves because parents are working or are not able to look after them and feed them. Such pressing needs have given rise to the formation of crèche associations. There are a total of five crèche associations. Some crèches are purpose-built and others are in shacks or rented four roomed township houses.

None of the crèches visited are funded or subsidised by the government. They are run as private concerns charging around R50 a month. In reality many families cannot afford to pay so some pay in instalments when they can. The Early Learning Project therefore raises money through jumble sales and donations to feed the children.

Women's Advisory Group

This is an emerging group. The women do not know yet how they will describe themselves but aim to provide a comprehensive advisory service to women, facing such problems as domestic violence. Many women who are beaten by their partners have no one to whom they can turn. I met such a woman who was advanced in her pregnancy, who described the abuse she endured. When an abused woman comes to the Centre the committee listens to her story. Four or five members of the committee meet with the partner to hear his side of the story and negotiate for a non-violent relationship. If the abuse continues the woman is advised to take legal action. In the meantime, she is assisted in moving into a women's refuge centre.

In a climate where competition for accommodation is rife, there are women who are made homeless as a result of their powerlessness. I joined a discussion about an elderly woman who was thrown out of her house by taxi men who wanted to use her home as a base in between taxi work. The women managed to get the woman back into her house but were uneasy about her safety and took turns to ensure that she was all right. In another case, the street committee, working with a council employee, sold a woman's house. The woman was a domestic worker in town and only came home at weekends. During the week another woman stayed in her house and looked after it. The street committee and their accomplice illegally determined that the woman had no right to the house and they sold it and divided the money between them. The dispossessed woman took her case to the Executive of the Women's Voice of Orange Farm and she got her house back. Why did the women not report the corrupt official?:

> We have approached him personally and he has denied any knowledge of this but we know that he is involved in these shady deals, but we can do little without evidence. What we are doing now is to collect a lot of evidence and in a very short time he will be out of that job. He is a real hindrance rather than a help to people looking for houses (Committee member, 1997).

The women are dismayed especially by crimes committed against pregnant women. They spoke of a group of young men who have slashed the torso of a pregnant woman to see the baby before it is born. It was not clear whether this was the work of a cult group or another manifestation of senseless violence. Whatever the motivation for these murders, the women in Orange Farm were determined to take steps to protect themselves. They formed groups in various parts of the township and it was to these groups that women reported what was happening in their areas. The group in turn informed the executive which is linked to various agencies which act accordingly to deter violence against women. The network was in itself protective in the sense that women were alerted to the dangers they faced, and they were on the look out for each other and came to each other's aid. Men are recognising that women have reached a point where they will defend themselves and that they are finding strength in collective action.

There are many other activities in Orange Farm which place women in the vanguard. They are involved in the welfare of the blind and partially sighted, people with disabilities, senior citizens, street children and abandoned babies. It is in the strategies they adopt as well as the boundaries they cross that capture domains that were once the preserve of men, which justifies the compelling conclusion that what I observed was women making 'herstory'. The networks they have created through the establishment of projects has given them confidence and mutual strength. When one group applies for funding or negotiates for a specific service, other groups write supporting letters stating how the proposed service would impact on the welfare of the community.

Although in areas like Orange Farm, the conditions under which people live, and against which women struggle, are far from satisfactory, there are glimpses of light and a hope that in the future things will improve. This is because women are determined to change their situations and those of their communities and are acquiring recognition. It is also because the government's economic policy is biased towards urban rather than rural development. Attracting foreign investment in the development of the infrastructure will benefit people in the townships. The RDP funds, which are supposed to be available to all are mainly targeting urban areas. Even independent funders find it easy to support projects in townships because of easy access geographically (there are roads and they can visit the projects themselves), and in terms of communication with the people involved (many people in townships speak English). Similarly, professional workers including those who work in the voluntary sector, are reluctant to take up posts in rural areas where there may be no roads, water, good sanitation, electricity, telephone, good schools or living wages. Even those who were born and brought up in rural areas tend to relocate in order to access these facilities in urban areas.

Women in Rural Areas

As a former resident of South Africa, I have not only travelled through but have lived and worked in many different rural areas. Under the apartheid regime all rural areas shared a common status. They were the dumping grounds for people cast as 'superfluous' to the needs of capitalism. The conditions that plagued many people and resulted in numerous deaths worsened between 1960 and 1982 when 1.2 million people were forcibly removed from their homes. A submission to the Truth and Reconciliation Commission concerning forced removals is uniquely revealing. It states that black people have rallied and made every effort to rebuild and restore their communities:

> Anybody who has seen the despair, the confusion and the powerlessness of people who had been summarily uprooted from their established homes and dumped in the veld cannot but be amazed that not only have many of them survived, but they have actually managed to re-build some form of community. They have not accepted, but they have come to terms with their fate. This is a tribute to their resilience, courage, ingenuity and the very humanness which was consistently denied by the apartheid regime.

The people at the centre of community building are women. My research turned to focus on the women of Vulamehlo, a rural area in the Umzinto magisterial district, 80 kilometres south of Durban in the KwaZulu-Natal province.

The area is typical of rural settings. There is no running water and women and children travel for hours to fetch water from rivers and springs. Boreholes are far from people's homes, many have run dry and infection from contaminated water is a real danger. Some people have built pit latrines but they are badly designed, unhygienic and are near houses and flies commute between toilets and houses. There is no electricity so women collect wood from shrub forests and carry it on their heads for miles. Those with money use one ring, paraffin primus stoves. Many homes are far from roads and it is not unusual to see a sick person being pushed in a wheelbarrow to a taxi stop. Some people described walking for over two hours to get to the nearest clinic. Even the community outstations visited by the mobile clinic once a month (and this is a recently instituted service), are still far from many people's homes and their infrequency means that people still need the services of the main clinic.

As in many other areas the clinic is overpowered by the number of people needing treatment. Accordingly staff decided to limit the clinics to 100 people a day. This means that people may travel long distances only to be told that they cannot be examined or treated. The clinic has maternity beds which are not used. It appears that the clinic has not enough staff, but it could also be that for many women the clinic is too far, lacks a welcoming atmosphere and that some women prefer to have their babies at home. The main problem is that there is no ambulance to take women experiencing complicated labour to hospital, and even if there was, many places do not have access to phones. Some places are so far from roads that the delivering woman is carried on a home made stretcher to reach the vehicle. The nearest doctor is at Umzinto, the nearest town, 35 kilometres away. Many people cannot afford the taxi fare and the doctor's fee. There are no employment opportunities in the area and men made redundant in the cities, sit around unoccupied. A gloomy reality within which women struggle to keep their families and community together. The situation was summed up in a report from a workshop attended by some women in this area before mobile clinics were introduced:

> The nearest clinic is at Jolivet, there is no ambulance to fetch the ill or pregnant women, no mobile clinic, no school nurse. Most mothers have their children immunised at the clinic. The mentally and physically handicapped people have no services. Some of the handicapped children are put in the crèches. Many children are born at home - it is too far and expensive to go to the hospital or clinic. In the gardens we grow mealies, madumbezi, sweet potatoes, cabbage and beans. There is little water and with no fences the cattle, goats and chickens, eat the plants. Some homes have a few fowls - they are used to eat, not to lay eggs. People fetch water from the Ndonyane and Mkhumbane rivers...

The women are assisted by two white women, Sr. Casian and Morley Bailey. Sr. Casian runs a weaving centre in which local women are employed. None of the women have academic qualifications. They are trained in the Centre to be dyers, spinners, designers and weavers. Women are paid according to their production. At the beginning the market was buoyant:

> We did a lot of wall hangings with African folklore designs and sold a lot of them to our German visitors (Sr Casian is German) as well as other people within South Africa. But not only is the market flooded with these products now but in times of inflation luxury goods like these are the first to be cut out in people's budgets. We now concentrate more on religious garments which are needed for mass celebration. We have

external markets in Zimbabwe, Maputo as well as internal ones in Portshepstone and Mariannhill. We have maintained the market for small orders for Germany, Austria and Switzerland. As a result all the looms are fully used and we are able to sell all that we produce (Sr. Casian, 1997).

The women in the Centre are breadwinners in their families. Some of them have seen their children through education to university level. All are able to feed their families and build homes for them. They all contribute to a saving scheme which directs profit to a bank to create a pension fund. When women leave the Centre they receive a lump sum, but many women stay for so long that the value of their lump sum is eroded by inflation. To reduce this possibility women are offered half of their money in the course of their employment to use as they wish, to build houses, buy furniture or pay for the education of their children. As Sr. Casian observed, there is more to this than the pursuit of economic ends:

> There is the human aspect, the spiritual development which is the motivation to continue to work. We start our work with a prayer and every week we have a bible study. We work as a community. We discuss our problems whether they are about work, home or children and we pray together. Tensions between us are resolved in the good old way where people say what they feel. The women have developed confidence, self worth, self esteem and creativity. The process of healing the ills inflicted by the system is achieved through creative involvement (Sr. Casian, 1997).

Siyabona (we see) Creative Learning Trust

The Trust is located in the Vulamehlo district within which is the Ndonyane Mission. The mission of the Trust is:

> ...to provide a comprehensive and holistic development programme to rural, marginalised communities, helping to upgrade living conditions while eliciting the creative potentials and strengths of individuals and communities (Siyabona leaflet).

Morley Bailey, one of the trustees was instrumental in setting up the Siyaphana Women's Movement.

Siyaphana (we share) Women's Movement

This movement is composed of 22 groups with a total of 500 women. The aim is to create a network of skilled rural women with the aim of actively improving their life conditions and those of their communities. Each group is represented in a committee that meets every month to discuss progress and problem solving.

The projects in which women are involved include sewing, knitting, candle-making, doll-making and gardening. Some of these activities existed before the establishment of Siyaphana, but bringing them under the umbrella of the Women's Movement has empowered women through working as a collective and has made available support and guidance which might not have been possible had they remained separate. The problems inherent in community projects are not different from those that exist in other parts of the country. One of these problems is the level of skill. In a sewing project for example, women may have the basic skill but the end product may be so poor that people would not be prepared to buy the finished article. We noted a similar problem with the Orange Farm women. In order to overcome this problem Siyaphana has brought in trainers to help improve the level of skill. The second problem, as always, is a viable market. Here again the organisation has been useful in forming a sewing club composed of trained women from each group which supplies a local school with uniforms.

Home Health Care

Siyaphana works closely with local heath institutions in developing a comprehensive district health care programme. Siyaphana's contribution is in three areas - training of traditional birthing assistants (TBAs), providing an educational health centre and facilitating a traditional healing project. Central to this contribution are community health workers (CHW), appropriately called in vernacular, Onompilo, (the healthy ones). We have already touched on the issues relating to the role of CHWs when we discussed the initiatives of NPPHCN. In the Vulamehlo area the need for the services of CHWs has been expressed by women in the Siyaphana group. Below we look at some of the activities that have involved the services of women working as community health workers.

Traditional Birthing Attendants (TBAs)

A large number of women in the Vulamehlo area deliver their babies at home. A conservative estimate has revealed that 45 - 60 percent of births in the area occur at home. In these births TBAs, with the skills passed on from generation to generation, play a central role. A study, conducted in the area in 1980/81 by researchers from King Edward VIII hospital in Durban, showed that contrary to the ridicule and dismissive attitude of some obstetricians, these TBAs have very useful advice and practices which must be encouraged. From the seventh month of pregnancy, for example, they advise the practice of coitus interruptus. The researchers quote the work of Naeye and Ross (1982) which has shown that the use of condoms in the third trimester reduces greatly the incidence of premature rupture of membranes, premature labour, incidence of abruptio placentae and perinatal mortality rate. The 'wise women of the village' do not use sophisticated methodologies but they know that sperms in advance pregnancy must not be allowed anywhere near the foetus.

In labour the researchers found that the TBAs encouraged women to be ambulant during the first stage and to adopt a kneeling position in the second stage of labour. They comment on this practice:

> There is now considerable evidence that the maintenance of an upright position in the first stage of labour is associated with less pain and more efficient uterine action, and hence a shorter labour. Our experience with the kneeling position in the second stage of labour shows that the adoption of this position also shortens the second stage and reduces pain. Encouraging mothers to be up and about during the first stage of labour and providing them with suitable diversions between checkings is elementary psychoprophylaxis which every hospital, including rural units, should use. Midwives and doctors working in rural areas should be taught to conduct deliveries in the squatting position so that this can be offered to women who prefer it as a matter of routine (Larsen et al, 1983 p.542).

This ancient wisdom merits sharing with all midwives and doctors so that they can offer this service to women who prefer it.

In calculating the expected date of delivery the TBAs in this study used a 36 week gestation period. They used the lunar cycle and delivery was expected anytime during the four weeks following the end of the ninth lunar cycle. The researchers confirmed that this method of calculation can be extremely accurate and they advised staff working with illiterate and semiliterate women to learn how to interpret it. This precludes staff concluding that 'all these women are ignorant and stupid'.

The researchers also found some practices which are potentially harmful. These included dietary taboos where pregnant women were not allowed to eat eggs, meat and milk from the family herd. This prohibition can grossly deplete the protein content in the diet leading to complications which include an increased incidence of intra-uterine growth retardation and perinatal death, particularly if the woman works for long hours and walks for long distances carrying heavy loads. I think it is important to view this prohibition in context. In the past, milk and meat from the family herd were easily available. To-day the situation is different. The prohibition remains but has little effect. These foods are not easily available to anyone. Even families which still have cattle, these do not provide protein on a daily basis. Prohibition or not, alternative sources of protein must be sought.

The Vulamehlo Experience The concerns expressed in the Larsen et al (1983) study re-surfaced among the Siyaphana members in the 1990s. They were concerned about poor facilities and limited knowledge in the areas of home deliveries, pregnancies and care for young children. They approached Siyabona Trust for assistance. This led to the development of a project in which 19 women in the Vulamehlo district were chosen by their communities to train in better birthing skills and improved health practices. The training of women was undertaken by a qualified nursing sister with community nursing experience. She trained in Kenya for six months in traditional birthing methods. Siyabona facilitated the training and support of TBAs linking them to the relevant clinics and hospitals to facilitate collaboration. The TBAs formed a committee which included representatives from health and education authorities and community leaders.

A survey was undertaken in 1997. Nineteen TBAs interviewed twenty women about their pregnancy, births and childcare. The information was assessed by hospital and clinic representatives and was used to inform the training programme. Training sessions were held in women's homes, health and education centres and in hospitals. Clinics and hospitals provided teaching material and birthing kits and offered access to observation and practical work. The trainees attended ante-natal clinics where they palpated pregnant women and listened to the foetal heart beat.

They visited labour wards and observed deliveries and the care given to the newborn.

The training that the women received was not intended to supplant traditional knowledge with conventional midwifery. It was to bring together good practices from both approaches and eliminate the harmful practices associated with pregnancy and childbirth.

At the end of the training the Vulamehlo district has TBAs to provide high-quality services and community training workshops whilst remaining linked to the clinics and hospitals for ongoing support and supervision.

In their communities the women have identified the need for general health care. Accordingly their training has included inputs to improve basic health care for individuals. A trainee stated:

> As soon as we learn about something, we put it into practice. Near me there is one elderly woman who lives by herself. She suffers from arthritis, she can hardly walk. I visit her in the evenings three times a week. I make a fire for her and wash her body with warm water and then rub her with embrocation. She looks forward to my visits and says that her pains are not as troublesome after the treatment.

Even if the 'embrocation' as a treatment was not effective, the attention and the company given to someone who spends evenings alone is enough to produce some sense of well being. Just to know that somebody cares is a tonic in itself. But the real pay off is that the community health worker is the link between the house bound elderly person and a variety of agencies including professional health workers.

In cases of diarrhoea and vomiting, whether it affects adults or children, the community health workers are there to initiate rehydration, a lifesaver in rural areas which are miles from conventional treatments such as drips and antibiotics. In some cases the patient improves without having to be taken to a clinic or hospital. There is no doubt that the TBAs have very important roles in the provision of primary health care in their communities.

The Community Health Centre

The Centre has been established as part of the comprehensive home-based health care programme. It is centrally based in the Ndonyane area and is therefore easily accessible to all in the Vulamehlo district. It is envisaged that the Centre will be used for a variety of activities: traditional birthing attendants will hold regular workshops on ante-natal and post-natal care, breastfeeding, immunisation and baby care; there will be trained AIDS volunteers hosting discussion groups in an attempt to combat the spread of AIDs. Young people will be involved in organising activities to raise AIDS awareness. Counselling will be given to AIDS sufferers and their families and advice will be given on the care of people with HIV/AIDS.

The Centre will be a focal point for health workers who are monitoring the medicine intake of TB sufferers as well as those who work with families on basic health care issues. There will be days when people come for health checks which will include screening for high blood pressure and diabetes. In addition the Centre will serve as a venue for talks and workshops on cancer awareness, eyesight and hearing problems. It will be used to tackle malnutrition in children below six years of age. Children suspected of being underweight will be weighed at regular intervals and food provided. All in all the Centre will be a forum for workshops and discussions on all health issues. It will be used by health professionals as a clinic. But the most novel contribution of the Centre is the role it gives traditional medicine in a place of healing.

Traditional Healing

Despite the proliferation of Western medicine in Africa, traditional healers have had an important role in the prevention and treatment of illnesses. In a world dominated by Western science and its leanings towards imperialism, indigenous knowledge on which traditional healing is based has been too easily ridiculed and dismissed as 'witchcraft' or 'black magic'. However, Mtshali, (1994) claims that the emerging political climate in South Africa has produced a marked change with regards to the rights of black people and respect for our culture e.g. in her thesis on indigenous knowledge, Mtshali notes that of the earth's 265,000 species of plants, Western scientists have only been interested in studying 1000 despite the fact that 40,000 are already used in traditional healing. But now there is a growing interest born out of the need to take account of the input of traditional healers in the delivery of primary health care since over 70 percent of black people consult traditional healers (Gumede, 1990).

That is not the only driving force in this shifting of view. The fact is that even those who are at times derogatory of traditional medicine recognise that the 'native doctor does sometimes work a cure where the efforts of European physicians have proved utterly unavailing' (Bryant, 1970). These cures have extended to black and white people. There are recorded examples of cases where Europeans were cured by traditional healers when Western medicine had failed. One instance was in the 19th century when a European woman, dying of sepsis was cured by a Bushman doctor. In Swaziland, a European doctor dying from dysentery was treated successfully by a traditional healer (Finch, 1989). African knowledge was not restricted to medical treatment, Finch provides many examples of traditional healers successfully applying surgical treatments. The most outstanding instance is that reported in the Edinburgh Medical Journal in 1884 by Felkin, a missionary doctor who witnessed a caesarean section performed by a Banyoro surgeon in Uganda in 1879. In his report Felkin included a detailed account of how the surgeon dealt with the third stage of labour and the suturing of the incision. The process revealed the depth of knowledge not only about anatomy and physiology but also anti-septic procedures. The thorn spikes that were used to close the incision were removed six days after the operation and when Dr Felkin left, eleven days after the operation, both mother and baby were well and the mother was up and about. Finch points out that at this point in the history of Europe caesarean sections were performed only to save the life of the baby. An operation to save both mother and child was unheard of nor were there any records of such an operation in any civilisations of antiquity. The instruments used and the procedures followed suggested the existence of a long practised skill by well-trained health experts:

> Not only did the surgeon understand the sophisticated concepts of anaesthesia and antiseptics but also demonstrated advanced surgical techniques. In his sparing use of the cautery iron, for example, he showed that he knew tissue damage could result from its overuse. The operation was without question a landmark, reflecting the best in African surgery (Finch, p.152).

These examples, which are not common knowledge to many, led Finch to conclude that Western 'scientific' medicine has its origin in the African continent. This may explain why, despite the proliferation of Western medicine, a large number of people in Africa still use traditional medicine. The knowledge has remained in the continent. It has been well tested and passed on from generation to generation but outside the framework of a health service loyal to Western medicine. This is not unique to Africa. The majority of the world's population 'receives its health care from traditional systems that are outside the formal health service' (Gorman, 1992). The impetus to Mtshali's thesis is the danger that environmental knowledge, of which medical knowledge is a part, will be lost as more and more young people lose links with their rural roots:

> This knowledge and the wisdom which accompanies it is kept in the minds of people, and is passed from generation to generation orally. The information needs to be retrieved, documented and disseminated before it disappears so that it can be included alongside the more usual 'scientific knowledge' in all types of education, namely, formal, and informal (Mtshali, 1994).

This concern is shared by the women in the Vulamehlo district. They go beyond the loss of knowledge through the severing of rural links in the younger generation at both physical and ideological levels. There is a growing number of people who use local herbs in order to make money. As many of them have no knowledge of the medicinal contents of what they sell to people, there is a strong probability that they do more harm than good. Others, still in pursuit of money, have become suppliers to urban-based traditional healers. They collect bags and bags of herbs and tree barks which they take to the city and sell to practitioners who determine what is of medicinal value. The damage to the environment is enormous because the money-motivated collectors, unlike the genuine traditional healers, have no knowledge of how to take from nature without harming the source of their supply. The genuine traditional healers, for example, know that when taking a bark from a tree one must not strip a total ring around the tree because that is harmful to the tree and will eventually kill it.

The major theme of Siyaphana is 'sharing' not just the material things but also the knowledge and the information. Amongst the community health workers are women traditional healers who are willing to share their knowledge with other women. The process is facilitated by a medicinal plant garden established in Chatsworth, a place outside Durban, by a man who wanted to save some of the species used in traditional healing from the onslaught of bulk collectors and destructive forest clearing. He wants to preserve plants for genuine healers who are allowed to visit and take what they need without destroying them. The traditional healers and the other TBAs share knowledge about what works and in what conditions. TBAs will be trained in the use of these herbs and in turn they will teach those who want to know how to use the herbs. People will be able to take cuttings of the plants in the health centre garden and plant them in their own home gardens. As a TBA said:

> I have been for some training already and I was quite surprised how much of what we dismiss as weed is very potent medicinally. Everywhere you go you will find a number of common weeds which when used at a certain stage in their growth span cure different diseases. Sometimes you find that the roots, the stem, the flowers and the leaves in one plant are all used to cure different conditions.

As we walked she picked different weeds telling me how they are used. We passed a guava tree and she picked some leaves from it:

> Five years ago I nearly died with stomach pains and diarrhoea. When I eventually got to the hospital the nurses assumed that I was going to die. They told me this when I recovered consciousness. Many people who went into hospital with me during that epidemic died. I think what saved me was my sister-in-law who poured jugfuls of water down my throat for hours before I was taken to hospital. Two weeks ago I had another attack of diarrhoea and the accompanying symptoms I had five years ago. I had my gallons of water near me, but in addition, I grounded the leaves of the guava tree, put them in a cup of water, strained them and drank the juice. By the end of the day I was as right as rain. I will share my experience with the rest of the group who will also try it to see if they have the same result. And that is how we collect our information, from experience. People, including traditional healers, can tell you what to use and for what. This is useful to ensure that those with little knowledge do not take death-causing herbs. But the real test of what works and what does not lies in us using the herbs rather than accepting on faith what others say.

Was it rehydration or the guava leaves that did the trick or indeed her belief in the potency of the guava leaves? This is a question that conventional 'scientists' go to extraordinary lengths to answer and in the process spend millions in experimentation. For this woman, the question is already answered by her own experience. But the TBA knows that until her cure has been tested and tried again by others she cannot conclude that guava leaves have curative properties. This is research at grassroots level. There are no trials on animals. With guidance from those who have more knowledge about which herbs are safe to take in what strength, the women in Vulamehlo are prepared to test out the medicine on themselves. They have the ability to be sensitive to the body's response to the ingested herb. Listening to the body's reaction is encouraged in the group discussions to which community health workers contribute.

I do not claim that this scenario depicts how traditional healing is conducted in general, not least as there are as many means of traditional healing as there are motives for doing it.

This project has adopted a radical approach in de-mystifying medical knowledge and de-centralising power that formerly belonged to 'traditional healers'. The women with the newly acquired skills are not setting themselves up as the new elite. They are sharing the information with people seeking assistance and encouraging people to take responsibility for their health instead of having 'professionals' telling them what to do and when to do it. This does not mean that trained traditional healers are redundant. They continue to have a specialist role as much as a specialist has in a hospital.

Healing occurs after damage. It consists of repairing tasks which would have lesser roles if a holistic approach to primary health care was a given encompassing the micro and the macro levels of health care. The women know that water, sanitation, housing, energy and employment, the macro factors in holistic health, are the responsibility of the government. What is within their power and that of their communities is the use of land in food production. Nutrition is the contribution they make in the level of health care.

The Crèche Project for pre-school Children

In the Vulamehlo district I interviewed a committee member involved in setting a crèche centre. She informed me that the ANC government encouraged communities to establish crèches in their areas. No resources were made available, instead, people were asked to offer their homes to be used as crèches:

> They said that it would only be for a short time and that money would be made available to build a proper crèche. My mother had died and her house was unused so I offered it to be used. The RDP gave us R5000 to buy food for the children. Three people worked in the crèche - one teacher, one support worker and one cook.

Money for the purpose built crèche eventually was made available through the links of Sr. Casian and Morley Bailey. Parents pay R25 a month, which many cannot afford. A staff member said:

> We divide whatever money is paid. Sometimes there may only be R100 or even less to divide among the three of us, and on other occasions we may have more. We cannot say at the moment that we do this job for money. But the children who come here do benefit because they get at least two meals a day which they would not get if they stayed at home.

In addition to payment parents were asked to give food donations. As voluntary contributions were uneven, staff used part of the grounds as a vegetable garden. A parent offered one of her fields for planting different foods but the problem at the time was that nobody had offered to till the soil and plant the seeds using oxen and there was no money for hiring a tractor. The staff believed that if they could have assistance in using the land the crèche would be on its way to self-sufficiency for most food that would be needed in the Centre.

The crèche used foods that were produced in the area instead of relying on expensive proteins like eggs, cheese and meat. In the vegetable garden staff used compost made from vegetable peelings. Apart from financial considerations - chemical fertilisers are expensive - this was a deliberate and informed decision to ensure that what the children ate was as nutritious as possible. The children using the crèche appeared healthy and alert. They were lively and happy looking compared to those who did not attend. As a grandmother noted:

> ...these children are quite bright. They are really clever. They sing songs and they can say some prayers as well. You should see the drawings they bring from the crèche. They are also polite when you talk to them. They ask you questions as if they are grown-ups. I have noticed this change not only with my grand daughter but also in the other children who use the crèche.

On another visit to Vulamehlo district I met with a committee member and crèche staff. The crèche had problems in getting money to buy food for the children. Was this a unique problem to this crèche or was this the situation with all crèches in the district? I asked Morley Bailey who was instrumental in setting up the other nine crèches which were distributed in different locations in the Vulamehlo district.

Table 6.2 Crèches in the Vulamehlo area

Crèche	Number of Children	Ward
Bambisanani	45	Bhobhobho
Inkanyisweni	34	Njane
Bekithemba	100	Mkhumbane
Siyakha	37	Mgangeni
Sizakancane	33	Bhobhobho
Umqangqala	35	Hlanzeni
Zamani	36	Hlanzeni
Sibongumusa	35	Hlanzeni

The problems faced by crèches were common. Many were run in homes with inadequate management, untrained staff and few resources. Committees from several crèches approached Siyabona for assistance. Their negotiations resulted in the establishment of an Umbrella Crèche Committee with the aim:

> ... to develop better management practices, establish a systematic training programme for staff and mothers of pre-school children and organise co-operative buying of food.

The committee also served as a channel for negotiating government subsidies. Whilst waiting for the subsidies the crèches survived on donations and moneys from trusts. Bringing crèches under one umbrella has ensured that whatever resources are available are shared. Donations and trust moneys, however, cannot be seen as long-term solutions. The Siyaphana committee is accordingly forward thinking in promoting the establishment of vegetable gardens in crèche grounds.

The Gardening Project

In the Vulamehlo district, the development of vegetable gardens is a legacy of the Nationalist government. People were encouraged to cultivate vegetable gardens that would provide them with produce through the year. Agricultural experts with assistants drawn from local communities were available to give guidance and advice. While people were not forced to join the scheme, if a plot was allocated and it was not used, it was re-allocated to someone else. Women are the cultivators in these gardens. They have not only benefited in terms of food for their families or a bit of money they make when they sell their surplus. As individuals they have been empowered by the knowledge they have gained through gardening and the successes they have had in producing high quality vegetables reflected in the many trophies they have won in regional agricultural shows. This has given them confidence and a belief in themselves.

Through my involvement these women formed links with a group in Liverpool which donated money to assist in the installation of a watering system which brings water pipes into the garden. The easy availability of water means that women can have a variety of vegetables right through the year and it also makes it easy to water each other's crops since all they need do is turn on the tap.

The process of empowerment for these women does not start and end in the vegetable gardens. They understand their position in the community and as a group they want to change it. This was an overarching theme in many of their workshops I attended. Whilst the women were pleased to have a chief who was a woman, a rare situation not only for their area but for South Africa, they were concerned that the tribal authority court over which she presided was dominated by men who made decisions without considering the issues faced by women. They wanted their voice to be heard at this level and they were asking the chief who inherited the all male cast, to ensure that in her next selection of council members women are fully represented.

In this chapter I asserted that black women have always been in the vanguard in providing services aimed at improving the health of their families and communities. In political struggles they have been over-represented in committees that dealt with housing, education, welfare and land, domains with known impacts on health. These are the same areas which concern women in the groups presented in this chapter. I have also asserted that in the process of meeting the needs of their families and communities women have made 'herstory' not only by crossing boundaries and challenging existing stereotypes about what is considered women's work but also by the strategies employed and the breaking of new grounds through projects undertaken.

The Learn and Earn project initiated by NCAW is a radical departure from the punitive practices characteristic of the justice system. Women accept the role of prison as a short-term measure in preventing people from committing crime. For long-term results they believe that the focus should be on enabling the individual offender to change his/her behaviour.

The Ikageng women are leading the way in implementing child-centred fostering. Foster parents are encouraged to move into the child's home rather than move the child from all that is familiar at a time when she/he is most vulnerable.

The introduction of practice nurses trained to diagnose and treat patients has been crucial in the provision of free services at primary health care level. Similarly, the introduction of community health care workers has been an important development particularly in the rural areas. Within NPPHCN, WHEP has played a leading role in moving these developments forward. The construction industry in which the Women's Voice of Orange Farm members are involved provides an example of how women are crossing boundaries and challenging stereotypes supported by patriarchal ideologies. These areas in which women are involved are not only making 'herstory' but they will have a tremendous impact in the development of South Africa. The breadth and the quality of these interventions indicate that black women in South Africa have an important role nationally and internationally.

References

Barnard, D. (1995), *Women's Organisations in South Africa: A Directory Programme for Development and Research,* PRODDER, July.

Bethlehem, M. (1997), *Makabongwe Amakhosikazi - Honour the Women*, National Council of Women of South Africa Conference.

Brayant, A.T. (1970), *Zulu Medicine and Medicine Men*, Gothic Printing Company Limited.

Finch, C.S. (1989),'The African Background of Medical Science', in Van Sertima, *Blacks in Science – Ancient and Modern*, Transaction Books.

Gorman, C. (1992), 'The Power of Option', *Times*, 30 April.

Gumede (1990), op. cit.

Hirschwitz, R. and Orkin, M. (1995) *Hearing the People – A National Health Survey of Health Needs*, NPPHCN, South Africa.

Larsen, J.V., Msane, C.L. and Monke, M.C. (1983), 'The Zulu traditional birth attendance – An evaluation of her attitudes and techniques and their implications for health education', *South African Medical Journal*, vol.63, pp540-543.

Mtshali, C.S. (1994), *Investigation of Environmental Knowledge among two Rural Black Communities in Natal*, unpublished Med thesis, Rhodes University South Africa.

Naeye, R.L. and Ross, S. (1982), Coitus and Chorisamnionitis: a prospective study, *Early Human Development*, vol.6, pp.91-97.

7   Care for Elderly People

In England, where black and ethnic minority elderly people have made their homes, research suggests that their needs at any level are not adequately met by service provision. A Birmingham study, conducted by Bhalla *et al,* (1981), revealed the poor health care received by black elderly people. Many received no treatment for eyes, ears, feet, or teeth and many remained isolated, unaware of services provided by social services, and they were not visited by social workers. A similar study was undertaken in Liverpool by Bonham *et al.* (1996). This study found a low up-take of services by black and ethnic minority elderly people despite the fact that they had high levels of unmet needs, a finding also evident in the use of hospital services (Torkington, 1991).

A well-rehearsed perspective on such evidence is the observation that black and ethnic minorities 'look after their own' because they have a strong kinship system. Although there are some people who do look after their elderly relatives we cannot assume that this informal care is available to all. We do not make this assumption about white elderly people.

Information collected in the course of this research suggests that in South Africa, although some elderly people are looked after by their families, others require a variety of support, including accommodation. This is reflected in the number of homes established by community voluntary groups. We visited some of these homes in the Gauteng and KwaZulu-Natal Provinces.

One of the community groups which recognised this need was the Ikageng Women's Group in the Gauteng Province. In the course of their work, members of the group were made aware of elderly people who had no one to care for them. In order to quantify the extent of the need, the women conducted a house to house research and as a result of the findings a decision was taken to establish a home. Money for the building was donated by church organisations and business companies. The Nationalist Government gave a small subsidy towards the running costs.

The home is in Soweto, one of the biggest townships in South Africa. It is a purpose-built Centre with sufficient pleasant grounds. It was well staffed and the residents were looked after and well occupied. A few stayed mostly in their rooms because of their poor health but the majority were active, taking part in a number of activities provided as part of the occupational therapy programme.

As with any service delivery, reliance on donations and people's good will is not the most effective way of providing a service. Fund raising for that level of operation needs full time experts. Financial insecurity inhibits long term strategic planning and creates insecurity and low morale among staff. It is in recognition of these factors that the trustees want to hand over the Centre to the government so that it can acquire mainstream funding. This proposal, a member of the Ikageng Women's Group informed me, has fallen on stony ground:

> The government does not want this type of home for elderly people. It says that in our culture elderly people are the responsibility of the community. They must be left in their houses and relatives and neighbours must look after them. We have done that. We have gone into houses where elderly people live alone, cleaned and fed them. But when we leave them at night criminals come in and not only rob them but also beat them up, rape them and in some instances, kill them. We have told them this. Frankly, I think the issue has little to do with culture, I think it has a lot more to do with money.

In the course of research this topic arose with a number of groups and individuals. In an area in Durban a man who has been campaigning for an old people's home in his community, confirmed the reluctance of the government to establish homes. But the reason, he stated, is not so much culture but finance:

> In our church we have discussed this with social workers and they have told us that the government says it has no money. The running costs for one person is R500 a month and the pension is below this amount. Many of the existing homes are being closed down because community groups are not able to maintain them. That is why the government is encouraging relatives and neighbours to look after elderly people in the community.

It is not only in relation to criminal strangers that elderly people are vulnerable. Abuse is also meted out by relatives, examples of which have been reported in the media. One elderly woman was left in a shack in the back garden whilst the grand children enjoyed the comfort of a big house. She was left dirty and soiled with just enough food to keep her alive. She was only cleaned and dressed on the day when she was taken to collect her pension which was immediately taken away from her. Fortunately neighbours contacted social workers who found a home for her, but others are not as lucky. In a group discussion a participant reported a recent death in her neighbourhood:

> We buried her two weeks ago but her body had been in the shed for two weeks before that. Her son and grandson have been taking all her pension and buying alcohol. This has been going on for a very long time. When she stood up to them and refused to give them the money, they threatened to kill her. We did not believe that they would do it. Then one day we did not see her around. We were told that she had gone to visit her relatives and would be back soon. After two weeks we became concerned, especially as some people were reporting a smell around the shed. Some people went into the shed and found the body and called the police. The post-mortem revealed that she was given an enema of undiluted jeyes fluid which filled her abdomen, and was locked-up in the shed where she was left to die. We are all still shocked about this.

Financial motives feature prominently in the abuse experienced by elderly people. Although not all elderly people are killed for their money, many are put under a lot of pressure to part with their pension. There are three main ways in which this pressure is exerted. The first occurs when relatives' demand pension money at knifepoint. They may accompany the elderly relative on pension day. They appear caring, loving and protective, only to take the money before the elderly person reaches home. Nurses working in casualty departments confirmed that some elderly people have injuries inflicted by their relatives because they refused to hand over their pensions. Can nurses intervene in this situation?

> We can if the person agrees. We get in touch with social workers who report the assault to the police and remove the elderly person to a home or keep an eye on her. But in most cases people do not want any action taken because they are frightened that their tormentors will kill them if they find out that they have been reported to social workers and the police. So we discharge them back to the same situation because we cannot act without their agreement and we know what they are saying is true.

The real problem here is that even when people report the attack to the police, very little is done to protect elderly people. This is demonstrated by an example from a rural setting. A grandson attacked his grandmother. When the neighbours heard the screams they rushed in to see what was happening. They caught the grandson and gave him a heavy beating, tied him up and called the police. The police arrived and took him away. Two days later he arrived home having been released. The grandmother was terrified and remains so in case he kills her:

> Calling the police was a mistake because they did nothing. He is away now working in town, but I am always frightened that when he comes home he will attack me again and this time he will kill me because I called in the police.

Six months after the incident two policemen called at the grandmother's house looking for the grandson because the case had to be taken to court. The grandmother chose not to proceed with the case and asked the police to abandon it. They told her she had to go to the magistrate to cancel the case. She refused and challenged them to arrest her:

> They cannot arrest criminals, let's see how good they are in arresting old women. I will not go to their court for anything. They have given me no protection.

The story illustrates the ineffectiveness of the police and the courts as deterrents and the reluctance of elderly people to report the ill treatment they receive.

The second form of pressure occurs when elderly people live in extended families and they are expected to contribute financially. Problems arise when the elderly person is left with R10 a month out of a pension of over R470. In some instances they are left with nothing as the nurses we interviewed testified:

> Relatives hire taxis and take their elderly relatives who are patients in our hospital to collect their pension. Some of them dress their grandmothers in mini skirts which suggests that the elderly person has no decent clothes of her own. When they bring them back the elderly people ask if we have kept any lunch for them. They don't even give them money to buy fruit or a drink. They bring them back into the ward penniless.

The third pressure hinges on the elderly person receiving the only source of income for a family of two or three generations. This concerns Lund (1995), when the government views increased spending on pensions as 'unproductive welfare spending'. She points out that two thirds of all black households are dependent on pensions for food, school fees, furniture and transport. She argues that reducing the pension will have layered impacts on poor black people (Lund 1995). Even though in this situation the money is used voluntarily for the love of the children and grandchildren, the physical consequences, in terms of reduced money for personal use including nutrition, are the same as if the money was forcefully taken from them. In the light of such realities the government must re-consider the welfare of elderly people in the community.

The abuse of elderly people by their family members is not unique to South Africa. As early as the 1970s and early 1980s, reports in both the United States of America and in the United Kingdom drew attention to an increase in the phenomenon. In 1981, for example, a report from a two year study by the Select Committee on Ageing of the United States House of Representatives concluded that:

> ... elderly abuse is far from an isolated and localised problem involving a few frail elderly and their pathological off-spring. The problem is a full-scale national epidemic which exists with a frequency that few have dared to imagine. In fact, abuse of the elderly by their loved ones and caretakers exists with a frequency only slightly less than child abuse in the United States (Kent County Council, 1989).

Statistics in Britain indicate that of elderly people, i.e. over 75, one in ten is at risk of abuse. Tales of abuse included:

> ... people being smothered to keep them quiet for a few minutes; the sexual abuse of an elderly woman by a lodger and the withholding of insulin from a diabetic person. Physical abuse, such as pulling and pushing, also occurs (Law, 1988).

These findings endorse earlier concerns expressed in the 1980s by social workers working with elderly people, e.g. Eastman (1982) highlighted and made visible the 'granny battering' syndrome providing concrete examples of abuse, which are not so different from findings in South Africa, i.e. Mrs N:

> ... a 74 year old widow who fractured her arm in a fall, is invited to live with her son and daughter-in-law, only to find she is confined to a small room upstairs. Anytime she attempts to go downstairs her daughter-in-law physically forces her back upstairs, often severely twisting the broken arm.

Another example concerns an elderly woman abused and beaten up by her married adopted son:

> When his business takes him to London he stays with his mother for two or three days. He expects her to prepare his meals and make his bed. The old lady is frightened of him and does not wish to take any action that could aggravate the situation.

In the United Kingdom our interviews with professionals who work with elderly people point to an increase in the abuse of elderly people following the 1990 National Health Service and Community Care Act. The Act introduced means testing for elderly people in city councils' care. The amount paid is based on a sliding scale. People with over £16,000 pay the full cost of care. If they have £10,000 they only pay the same amount as their pension and the city council pays the rest. If they have no savings but own a house, then they have to sell the house to pay for their care. These inroads into what family members may regard as their inheritance impacts negatively on elderly people, as one informant explained:

> Sometimes relatives will manage in a situation where they might have given up if it had not been for the fact that money will have to be paid if the elderly person was taken into care. Some people are honest and up-front about this. They will tell you that the old person's money is needed to keep the other members of the family. Some hide the fact that the house is owned by the elderly person and say that 'oh mum always said that the house will be mine' or they fiddle the system and make out that the house was signed over to them (Social worker, 1998).

When money is the issue relatives may endure very stressful situations which can lead to the abuse of the elderly person. Professionals sometimes know that an elderly person is abused but they cannot do anything because there is no legislation, other than the Mental Health Act, which gives them power to remove the elderly person from an abusive situation:

> If the elderly person is not mentally ill they have a right to decide what to do. If we detain them their relatives have a right to take them back. A lot of elderly people stay in abusive situations for a variety of reasons – they may be frightened of the abuser, they may not want to go to a home, they may be physically disabled or they may be used to the abusive situation. But we are powerless under the existing legislation. It is very frustrating when you know that the elderly person is abused and you can do nothing about it (Social worker, 1998).

The ill treatment of elderly people is not confined to the ranks of the unemployed. In families with employed professionals, many of them educated by the elderly parent, there is evidence of abuse. In South Africa we were told of an elderly woman whose family dispensed with the services of a domestic helper and forced the feeble grandmother to cook and clean for them. In another case the grandmother was left alone the whole day and guarded by dogs to ensure that no one came in to see the conditions under which she lived. Church members and other relatives could not go pass the dogs, nor could social workers. The son made it clear that he did not want anyone seeing his mother and that was the sole purpose of keeping vicious dogs on guard when he was at work. It is most unlikely that either of these people had access to their pension money.

The problem of elderly abuse which South Africa shares with other countries is a reality which will not go away. It is unrealistic and contrary to its own constitution for the government to endorse family and neighbourhood care when there is enough evidence to suggest that many elderly people are facing abuse within their families and communities. Nor is it acceptable to point to inadequate resources. It is a question of priorities. The number of old people's homes, which were built without government support during the apartheid regime, suggests that there are many people and organisations who see the need and are therefore prepared to contribute towards meeting that need. Maybe homes are not the answer. In the British situation there is evidence to suggest that being in an old people's home does not protect people from abuse. The South African government needs to consult and discuss with groups and elderly people themselves in order to find a way of providing safe, comfortable and valued accommodation and support.

The South African government has introduced free services for elderly people. Whilst this is welcomed by all, it cannot wipe out diseases which are the consequences of years of poverty and health undermining patterns of work. Many black elderly people suffer from various forms of dietary deficiencies that leave them open to an array of infections. It is a major problem that services such as the provision of spectacles and hearing aids are not free and not affordable by many elderly people. In rural areas elderly people, even if they had the money, have no access to such services.

Abuse in any shape or form is a serious threat to the health, well being and lives of many elderly people. Unless we die prematurely, all of us will experience old age. The following poem by an anonymous 'crabbed old woman' should alert each of us to our vulnerability and propel us to make adequate provision for elderly people.

Crabbed Old Woman

What do you see nurses, what do you see
What are you thinking when you look at me?
A crabbed old woman, not very wise
Uncertain of habit, with faraway eyes
Who dribbles her food and makes no reply
When you say in a loud voice, 'I do wish you'd try'
Who seems not to notice the things that you do
And forever is losing a stocking or shoe
Who, unresisting or not, lets you do as you will
With bathing and feeding, the long day to fill
Is that what you're thinking, is that what you see?
Then open your eyes, you're not looking at me.
I'll tell you who I am as I sit here so still
As I move at your bidding, as I eat at your will
I'm a small child of ten with a father and mother
Brothers and sisters who love one another
A young girl at sixteen with wings on her feet
Dreaming that soon now a lover she'll meet
A bride soon at twenty – my heart gives a leap
Remembering the vows that I promised to keep
At twenty-five now I have young of my own
Who need me to build a secure happy home
A woman of thirty my young now grow fast
Bound to each other with ties that should last
At forty my young now will soon be gone
But my man stays beside me to see I don't mourn
At fifty once more babies play round my knee
Again we know children, my loved one and me
Dark days are upon me, my husband is dead
I look at the future, I shudder with dread
For my young are all busy rearing young of their own
And I think of the years and the love I have known
I'm an old woman now and nature is cruel
'Tis her jest to make old age look like a fool
The body it crumbles, grace and vigour depart
And now there's a stone where I once had a heart
But inside this old carcass a young girl still dwells
And now and again my battered heart swells.

I remember the joys, I remember the pain
And I'm loving and living life over again
I think of the years all too few – gone so fast
And accept the stark fact that nothing can last
So open your eyes, nurses, open and see
Not a crabbed old woman – look closer – see me.

(Anonymous)

References

Bhalla, A. and Blakemore, K. (1981), *Elders of the Minority Ethnic Group*, AFFOR, Birmingham.

Boneham, M. A., Williams, K.E., Copeland, J.R.M., MCKibbin, P., Wilson K., Scott, A. and Saunder, P.A. (1996), 'Elderly people from ethnic minorities in Liverpool: mental illness, unmet needs and barriers to service use', *Health and Social Care in the Community, vol.5, No.3*, pp.173-180.

Eastman, M. (1982), 'Granny battering: a hidden problem', *Community Care*, 27 May.

Kent County Council (1989), *Practice guidelines for Dealing with Elder Abuse*, Social Services Department.

Law, J. (1988), 'Elderly Care: Houses of Horror', *Community Outlook*.

Lund, F. (1995), 'A Source of Household Security – The Social Security System and Budget', *Critical Health*, No.47, pp.47-52.

Torkington, N.P.K. (1991), *Black Health: A Political Issue*, Catholic Association for Racial Justice and Liverpool Institute of Higher Education.

8 Black People and Mental Illness

In the house in which I lived in Cape Town a group of church women met every Wednesday between eight and ten o'clock in the evening. When I was free I joined them. In between prayers and singing they exchanged information about their various activities during the week. Some of the white women visited a local mental hospital. They talked about the poor conditions in the wards. Nothing was done to stimulate patients, they were given drugs which left them half asleep most of the time. If this was the situation for white patients what was the position with regard to black patients?

The Historical Perspective

In South Africa people with mental health problems were left to the mercies of privately owned institutions. The most infamous was the Smith Mitchell and Company Limited of Johannesburg which was a profit making organisation which worked in collaboration with the Department of Health (Seedat, 1984).

The company was paid a fee, per patient, per day. Conditions in these private settings were acknowledged to be worse than those in the state institutions which were predominantly used by white patients. The private institutions were situated in old mine compounds with wire fences and wire mesh windows. Patients slept on grass mats which they made. These were spread on a cold cement floor. There was no bed linen or toilet paper. Patients were assaulted or witnessed assaults on other patients. Food was so bad that at one stage patients rioted in protest. Many patients died because they lacked medical care during their stay in these 'compounds'.

The conditions in the Smith Mitchell institution created a government scandal when the press exposed the situation to the public. The journalist who accidentally entered the institutions described them as 'the South African version of Dickensian workhouses'. Seedat estimates that at the time the company was accommodating 10,000 black patients, the majority of them involuntarily, several white, coloured and Indian patients. The government responded with a Mental Health Amendment Act which prohibited anyone who had not been given permission by the Secretary of State from entering and taking photographs in these mental health institutions. Those who contravened the Act could face a R1000 fine or imprisonment with no option, or both. This was done, the government proclaimed, to protect the privacy of mentally ill people. But those who understood the government of the day knew that the real reason for the Act was to stop public discussion and criticism.

In 1978 the South African Government, with the Smith Mitchell Company, invited the American Psychiatric Association to send a delegation to investigate mental health conditions in South Africa. The Association confirmed the findings of the press. Subsidies for white patients were R7 a day and only R1.50 for black people. The delegation concluded that:

> ...there is good reason for international concern about black psychiatric patients in South Africa. We found unacceptable medical practices that resulted in needless deaths of black South Africans. Medical and psychiatric care was grossly inferior to that of whites. We found that apartheid has a destructive impact on families, social institutions and the mental health of black South Africans. We believe that these findings substantiate allegations of social and political abuse of psychiatry in South Africa (Seedat, pp.52-53).

The conditions in state mental hospitals were no better for black people. There was a huge difference between white and black provision. Black patients were transferred to the private sector without receiving adequate medical and psychiatric assessments. Bed occupancy was 2.5 per 1000 whites and 0.8 per 1000 blacks which included Africans, Indians and Coloureds.

The situation had not improved in the 1980s. In 1982 Baragwanath General Hospital admitted at least ten mentally ill people a day. At the time the hospital had only two psychiatrists who held consultation sessions one day a week. There was only one psychologist for the hospital who saw patients four times a week. There were no special facilities for the mentally ill. In most cases they were put in wards with patients who were physically ill and to control them, they were tied to the beds. They had labels pinned on their gowns so that whoever met them wandering about would know that they were mentally ill and return them to the ward.

Seedat informs us that in 1982 none of the psychiatrists who treated Africans could speak any African language never mind understand or respect African culture. There were only eight black psychiatrists - seven Indian and one Coloured. At the time one African was being trained at the Medical University of South Africa (MEDUNSA) in Bophuthatswana, and another was due to begin training in Hillbrow hospital in 1983. All this was in the 1970s and 1980s. Has anything changed? Not according to the Mental Health and Substance Abuse Committee (MHSAC) which produced its Report in January 1996 on 'Human Rights Violations and Alleged Malpractice in Psychiatric Institutions'.

Mental Health in the 1990s

The Mental Health and Substance Abuse Committee was set up to investigate malpractice by managers and staff and the violation of fundamental rights of mentally ill patients in 32 hospitals in different parts of the country. The Committee investigated conditions and practices in three types of accommodation:

- publicly maintained psychiatric institutions;
- state subsidised institutions administered by Life Care Holdings;
- psychiatric wards in general hospitals.

The criteria used to assess mental heath provision in these institutions were the size of the wards; the physical state of the ward including bed linen, clothing for the patients, toilets, washing and bathing facilities; food; medical care; administration and the general treatment of patients.

The findings of this study revealed that the standard of care in institutions that were formerly used by black people was much lower than in those used by white patients in terms of the structure of the buildings, staffing and resources. In the majority of hospitals patients were paid a pittance for the work they did. In some institutions patients were given tobacco as an incentive to work, disregarding the damaging effect smoking has on health. Typically institutions were found to be overcrowded and short staffed, which in some instances led to the physical abuse of patients. However, this was difficult to verify because staff protected each other when allegations were made. The Committee concluded somewhat equivocally that:

...the conditions in most prisons around the country are better than those existing in some psychiatric hospitals. Some patients' deaths in psychiatric hospitals can in a sense be attributed to the conditions under which patients are being kept (MHSAC, 1996 p.80).

The Committee attributed malpractices and human right violations in mental institutions to the legacy from the apartheid system. They pointed out that inequalities in treatment and in the allocation of resources is 'the life-blood of management and administration'. Racism remains central stage in psychiatric institutions. There is protective legislation which criminalises any publication in relation to hospital affairs. This ensures that violations of human rights are unchallenged and as a result 'culprits have committed gross abuse on patients with impunity and with certainty that they will get away with it'. There is inefficiency at hospital board level and there is no accountability of those who certify patients. As well as the abuse of certification, there are no proper prescription guidelines, and widespread malpractices in medication lead to the use of cheap psychotropic drugs with harmful side effects. The use of ECT is unregulated and alongside limited community involvement a picture emerges of the multifactoral nature of system abuse:

> The limited and in many cases total absence of the involvement of communities and families of patients, also contributes to malpractices such as unwarranted continued institutionalisation. The prevailing no-discharge system at most of the hospitals can be attributed to little or no involvement of families and communities (MHSCA, pp.81-82).

The Committee identified some recommendations to improve the situation of mentally ill people. It stressed the importance of radical change in community attitudes towards mentally ill people as this gets in the way of communities concerning themselves with the welfare of mentally ill people. People with mental illness are seen as a burden and their institutionalisation necessary and a needed relief. Mental health institutions should be small and of manageable size. They must be located where they are easily accessible to relatives in order to facilitate and maintain links between patients, their families and communities:

- codes of practice must be laid down in order to protect the human rights of mentally ill people;
- there must be a Charter for patients' rights in which patients and their families are made fully aware of their rights;

- there must be regular inspection of the institutions by an independent panel composed of user representatives, leaders of local communities and professionals in health in general and psychiatry in particular;
- there must be clear procedures for complaints without fear of victimisation;
- there must be an ombudsman to investigate each complaint thoroughly;
- if abuse is confirmed, culprits should be prosecuted;
- certification should be the last resort if voluntary admission is not possible.
- the transfer of patients into private contract hospital must only be done by state doctors who should also review the progress of such patients and consider their release into the community;
- any patient who is kept involuntarily for over a year must be referred to the ombudsman;
- the role of the ombudsman must also be directed at the conditions in the mental institution;
- the number of patients in any given hospital must not exceed 400;
- a minimum of staff-patient ratio must be laid down to ensure that work is uniformly distributed among all professionals;
- hospital buildings must facilitate rehabilitation;
- disparities between institutions should be addressed urgently;
- staff training and development must be promoted to upgrade the standard of care and to introduce positive staff attitudes towards patients;
- community education programmes must be established to challenge the stigma of mental illness in the community and to facilitate the integration of mentally ill people into their communities;
- the Government must consider the decentralisation of the budget as centralised planning and budgeting is restrictive and does not allow local managers discretion.

This array of recommendations is impressive. Has much been achieved in terms of re-shaping provision? I addressed this question to people who worked with people with mental health problems.

One of the people I interviewed was a psychiatrist who has worked in all Johannesburg's psychiatric acute care units. She knew their bed occupancy, routine care and medication regimes. She was aware of the differential diagnosis between black and white patients. She argued, for example, that eating disorders are as common in black middle class young women as they are among their white counterparts. The perceived discrepancy is a question of diagnosis rather than the absence of this condition in the black population. She drew attention to obsessive compulsive disorders where a person is imprisoned by the compulsion to do things repeatedly, e.g. teeth brushing is not stopped even when the gums and teeth are damaged. Some people cannot go to work because they feel they have to keep washing their hands and water bills soar. In the mid 1980s and early 1990s this was not seen as a 'black disorder'. Black patients were simply defined as 'psychotic'.

The psychiatrist worked in a general hospital with 155 psychiatric beds. They admitted acute patients for short periods only because of bed shortages. This limited admission was a real burden to families who did not know how to cope with their mentally disturbed relatives when they were prematurely discharged from hospitals:

> You are either in hospital or suffering with your family. There are no support systems or drop-in centres or anything. I think if this is the situation in Johannesburg, I would think this is also the case in the whole country. I believe one man has set up some day care service in Cape Town. But I don't know a lot about it except that it is not a government scheme. There are community clinics of course, but all that happens in those clinics is that patients are given their medication and nothing else.

One project had been set up for the relatives of patients with schizophrenia. The money and the programme for the project was provided by Lundberck Pharmacy and was facilitated by the psychiatrist. Relatives attended one and a half sessions a week for eight weeks. The aim was to inform the families of patients with schizophrenia about the condition in the hope that the understanding would enable them to cope with the needs of their mentally ill relatives. Understanding is fine but people also wanted support and solace. They needed supporting structures in the community which will assist in the care of mentally ill people, structures that help not only in giving medication but which attempt to rehabilitate people back into the life of their communities.

Only two clinics had any form of rehabilitation. These were introduced by occupational therapy students on training placements. They raised money to buy material for activities. Patients who came to the clinic paid R5 a month and they got lunch and coffee:

> One of these clinics is doing really good work. Patients have an outing once a week. They choose where they want to go. Local transport is used

and they take packed lunch with them. The occupational therapy students are really good. They do things with people which help them to re-integrate back into society. What they do should be available to all mentally ill patients as a form of rehabilitation.

In her own hospital there was a team of a psychiatrist, psychologists, social workers, occupational therapists and nurses. They provide services which included counselling. However, the numbers of patients and the relative scarcity of beds meant that patients are not kept long enough to benefit from what was provided. If the situation was bad for adult patients, it was worse for children. There were no special beds for mentally ill children. What was available were day centres for assessment, treatment and follow-ups. The situation for children with learning disabilities was as bad. Very few were detected at an early age. The familiar pattern was for such children to be left in ordinary schools, labelled as 'difficult to teach' or 'naughty'. When they were about 12 years old, and it became obvious that they had learning disabilities, special schools refused to accept them because they were too old. They then joined the growing army of children who roamed the streets, some of whom were labelled mentally ill. There was an urgent need for improved communication between welfare, education and health departments and to increase provision for children with learning disabilities. Soweto, with its population of over two million people had only two special schools.

The inadequate provision for mentally ill people in the public sector has stimulated the private companies to establish facilities for the treatment of mentally ill people. Some of these are units in existing private hospitals but others are autonomous hospitals and clinics. I visited one of these in the Western Cape Province and had an interview with some members of staff.

Private Health Care for Mentally Ill People

The private hospital I visited is in Cape Town. It was set up in 1980. It is a 60 bed general psychiatric institution with 24 nursing staff, nine administrators, six general assistants and one laundry person. The cooking and the serving of food is in the hands of a private company which produces a weekly menu from which patients choose what they want. The clinic is clean and comfortably furnished. Smoking is only permitted in the smoking lounge and outside. Although some bedrooms may be shared by more than two, the norm is for two patients to share a room except for those with eating disorders where a group of four or five may share a bedroom for observation purposes. The Centre has three units: chemical dependency, eating disorders and psychotherapy.

Chemical Dependency Unit

A leaflet on the aims and objectives states that this unit:

> ...provides an in-patients drug and alcohol rehabilitation programme. It is an intensive programme aimed primarily at penetration of the denial system that keeps the alcoholic and addict locked into their disease. The focus is on the harmful consequences of the disease.

The programme has three phases. A detoxification phase if required, an intensive two - three weeks residential and a weekly aftercare phase for a minimum of eight sessions. Although the therapy is usually conducted in a group setting, each patient is assigned an individual counsellor. In order to encourage family members to take part in the recovery process, they are invited to participate in joint sessions during the course of the three residential weeks. The eight session aftercare programme consists of a weekly evening support group with an option to have a 'life skills' class. Patients are encouraged to have an active participation in Alcoholics Anonymous (AA) and Narcotics Anonymous (NA). The unit has a team of four counsellors, a full-time doctor and has the backing of the full complement of nursing personnel.

Eating Disorders and Adolescent Unit

The unit was added to the Centre in 1993 for the treatment of Anorexia Nervosa, Bulimia and Obesity. When it was opened it took in four or five patients but that number has increased to between 10 and 15 patients. Most of the patients are female, white and come from middle-class professional families where at least one of the parents is a doctor. The psychiatrist only recalled one male patient in all that time and no black patients. The goal of the unit is to:

> ...empower patients to take responsibility for themselves by moving beyond feelings of shame, isolation and helplessness to discover their values, emotions and needs. To accomplish this the unit provides each patient with the opportunity to participate in respectful, open and honest

relationships which support individuality and which work toward developing competency (Clinic leaflet).

A clinical psychologist who heads the unit believes that for most people treatment should initially be on an out-patient basis and that to be admitted the duration of the illness should be at least six months. Those who have had the condition for less than that period should only be considered for admission 'if their disorder is of severe intensity (physically and/or psychologically) and rapidly becoming chronic'. Conditions such as depression, anxiety, adjustment and conduct disorders are some of the reasons considered for an in-patient programme even if the patient has not manifested the illness for six months.

The in-patient programme is implemented by a specially trained team consisting of a clinical psychologist, primary therapists, an occupational therapist, movement therapist, a creative arts therapist, a social worker, a registered dietician and a team of four specially trained nurses. The clinical team is supported by a consulting team of medical specialists who maintain regular contact with the staff and the patient community. Admissions are relatively short and are followed by out-patient sessions. Treatment is based on individual, group and family therapy. For individual psychotherapy each patient has one session a week provided by a primary therapist who has a master-level degree. Only under special circumstances does a patient get more than one session a week.

For many patients who come into the programme, some of their problems lie in family relationships. This is especially the case 'where there has been serious physical and/or sexual abuse as well as in cases of a bad divorce'. The value of family therapy here, states the leaflet:

> ...is to help each patient's attempt to rework their relationship with family members, to evaluate the limitations of those relationships and to set realistic expectations. Joint sessions sometimes resolve conflict that has been continuing for years, allowing the daughter or son to have a relationship with each parent without a feeling of betrayal.

In a family support group which is usually available in the Centre, families get the opportunity to share their concerns, compare and attempt to solve together some of their common problems. The group is open to any family member who wishes to attend. Such family involvement augments the individual family therapy provided during admission, and acknowledges the family's potential as a primary resource for healing.

During the in-patient period patients attend a minimum of 20 group sessions during which individuals are given the opportunity to learn to confront and express their thoughts and judgement on a variety of subjects including 'self-esteem, assertiveness, sexuality, body image, nutrition and other educational themes'. The sharing validates each patient's individual experience as well as giving support to individual differences.

The clinic is aware of numerous studies which have indicated that the majority of women with an eating disorder have been sexually abused in the past. In order to support such patients the Centre has a Women's Empowerment Group. The group is facilitated by two therapists with special training. In the group women share their experiences with others, often for the first time, and explore the relationship between abuse and reactions to life events and stages.

The minimum period of admission is four weeks but some patients may need more than this in order to make more significant progress emotionally and physically. The discharge of a patient is a gradual process moving from in-patient to a weekly out-patient attendance. As patients progress they begin to attend selective programmes relevant to their needs. These may be in the area of supervised meals, group therapy or body image. As a day-patient, attendance does not usually exceed five hours a day. All patients are finally expected to enter into a follow-up therapy with either their own therapist or with a hospital one. They are also expected to attend a follow-up support group which runs one evening a week.

The Psychotherapeutic Unit

The unit is for general psychiatric patients. The aim is to enable patients to find ways of coping with their problems through gaining insight into their feelings, attitudes and behaviour. Treatment is based on group work. The Centre does not deal with patients who are under Section. Patients who injure themselves are immediately transferred to another hospital which deals with severely ill patients. Because of this arrangement drugs are used sparingly. Although some patients have Electro-Convulsive Therapy (ECT), one to one and group counselling are the norm in the treatment of patients.

As a private service, the Centre charges fees which fall within the recommended scale determined by the Representative Association of Medical Schemes. In 1997 psychiatric patients in a general ward with overnight stay paid R359 a day and without a night over-stay, R249. Out-patient facilities worked out at R124.70 a day. These charges excluded medicine, the use of specialised equipment and anaesthetic agents. The fee for ECT, for example, was R181.50 and to monitor a patient who had had this treatment cost R56.48. Patients on Medical Aids had these charges paid by their schemes, but they had to make sure before admission that their benefits included psychiatric care. Some schemes did not include alcohol and drug dependency and even those which did would only pay for up to three weeks. Many of the patients therefore were private in which case the psychiatrist observed, 'they must pay up-front before we admit them, a deposit or the full amount in some cases'.

Although the work of the above Centre may meet the needs of its users it is difficult to see how the model can be replicated in the whole of South Africa. It is based on profit making which means that the high charges paid exclude millions of people who are in desperate need of mental health services. Another limitation is the exclusion of people with severe symptoms of mental disturbance. Patients who attempt to injure themselves, for example, are transferred to other hospitals. A state service cannot be this selective because it provides for all, irrespective of the degree of the illness. Finally, and perhaps more importantly, mental illness is not just an individual or a family problem. It may manifest in the individual but its roots are in the society in which the individual lives, and so must be its treatment. Mental health provisions must not only be based in the areas where patients live but must involve communities in the process of re-integrating patients back into their communities. Treatment and rehabilitation must take place within a network which links all structures and services which impact on a patient. Just a few examples to illustrate this point. The Inkageng women, whose activities were discussed earlier, campaigned for a disability grant for a brother and a sister who were defined as mentally ill. The grant not only gave them independence but motivated them to get casual employment which has ensured integration into their community. Apart from providing a livelihood, employment is a powerful symbol of identity. It is important that employers in the public, private and voluntary sectors are drawn into the network with work schemes for people recovering from mental illness. However, all of this will need substantial understanding and changes of attitude towards those affected by mental illness. This is the role of education in its broadest sense.

It is important that mental health provision does not only deal with the presenting patient, but that it links with other structures that will look at the background of patients and respond to the difficulties uncovered. Many mentally ill people in townships with whom the Inkageng women have been involved, are homeless and hungry and for many this may be the cause of mental illness.

The Voluntary Sector

The information gathered during this research suggests that there has been little work done by the voluntary sector to address the needs of mentally ill people. The two services discussed below are pioneering initiatives in Cape Town.

COMCARE

COMCARE was set up to work with people who had been diagnosed and treated as schizophrenics. The history goes back to 1986 when two white families were faced with the problem of accommodation when their children were discharged from hospital. The facilities and the care in the Home to which they were discharged were not suitable, stated one of the parents. The two families put money together and with the help of a bond (mortgage), bought a house and advertised for a house-mother. This was not an easy start as there were quite a lot of teething problems:

> Once we had the house and made some alterations, we advertised for a house mother. We got one quickly but she was alcoholic and so we could not really keep her. We had to look for another. Then nobody came forward to use the house even though we advertised. Even the daughter of the family with whom we bought the house refused to come. For six months our son was the only one who lived in the house with a house-mother, but by the end of the year there were five people in the house.

The patients who lived in this house remained stabilised with no relapses. As people became aware of its success the demand for more facilities increased. In 1991 the founders took out another bond and bought a second house. In the same year COMCARE, a charitable trust was established to 'maintain facilities and programmes in the community for the persistent, severe and prolonged mentally ill people in the Western Cape Region'. The main objective of the trust is to:

> ...establish group homes in the community through the raising of funds. These homes will vary in the degree to which the residents would require supervision from fully supervised on the one hand and unsupervised on

the other. These homes will be for those individuals without any financial resources (COMCARE leaflet).

Besides providing accommodation, the Trust was raising awareness about the positive effects a caring and befriending community could have in the lives of people after they had been discharged from hospital. It played an informative role to local and central government, the media and general public about the needs of mentally ill people.

COMCARE was run by a combination of paid staff and a group of volunteers. There was a full-time secretary, a full-time social worker, a part-time chief executive and house-mothers in various homes. Some volunteers were trustees and others were involved in the management structure within which they monitored the functioning of the group homes. There was a group of about 100 families which met once a month to provide support and share ideas and difficulties in coping with a relative with mental illness. I interviewed one member of the group who expressed the dilemma of parents whose children had mental illness:

> The major problem is trying to cope with the illness and the personality. The behaviour can be so annoying and frustrating that one becomes really angry. You have to pull yourself up and remember that this person is ill and that maybe the behaviour is linked to the illness. But sometimes you think it is just their personality and they are just manipulating the situation. A lot of us worry about how one can tell which is which.

At first the group was not recognised by hospitals or the Department of Health, but later was accepted as a needed community facility. Members go all over the world attending conferences and collecting information which enhances the work of COMCARE. They are now affiliated to similar organisations in different countries. At the time of the research there was a move to involve users in the international link by establishing a pen-friend scheme with users in group homes in America.

I visited some group homes. The houses were ordinary homes in a residential area. In one of the houses there were six residents, four women - one coloured and three white, two men - one black and one white. I asked the housemother who had been there for more than three years, and described herself as 'coloured', if there were any problems arising from this racial mixing:

> ...no not at all. They get on very well. They sit together, eat together and sometimes go out together. To-day for instance, a sister of one of the

residents is having a birthday party, and we have all been invited, so we are all going.

The routine was supervised by the housemother who cooked the evening meal. Residents prepared their own breakfast and had their lunch at Fountain House, a local day care centre to which the Trust pays R7 a day, per member. They cleaned their rooms, washed dishes and generally kept the house tidy. They had to be out of the house between 9.00 am and 1.00 pm. Although they were encouraged to attend the Centre, they were not restricted from going anywhere else in that period. It was the responsibility of the housemother to see that the routine was adhered to:

> My relationship with the residents is good. None of them show any racism towards me. I am quite strict and consistent with them. I see to it that they wash themselves and get dressed properly before they leave the house, that they take their medication and that they are out of the house at the stipulated time. Of course there is some flexibility but the norm is that they are out for at least four hours so that they mix with the outside world. I let them know that no is no. I am the housemother and I am paid to do a job.

All the houses had someone who came to do washing, ironing and cleaning and it was the housemother who ensured that all this was done efficiently. In general the housemother was committed to the job and enjoyed it, but felt that there was a lot of responsibility and stress and 'one is engaged in solving problems that arise between residents'. Even though there was a cleaner, the housemother still had to do 'the finishing touches'. She also went with the residents on various trips and organised evening games with people in other houses in the area. Her only concern was that her salary did not match the amount of work and the responsibility it entailed.

In the other house I visited the housemother was a black woman. She had the same kind of duties and responsibilities. There were six residents, all men - four white and two 'coloured'. The mother felt that there was some resistance to her supervisory role. The residents were reluctant to clean their rooms or wash dishes and at times she ended up doing the work and getting them breakfast. The relationship between her and the residents was nevertheless friendly except for one man who exhibited racist behaviour especially when he was going through a rough period in his illness.

COMCARE was aware of the pivotal role housemothers had within the organisation. Although some of them did not sleep in, they still spent a lot of time with the residents and they were on the spot to notice any change in the condition of patients. Housemothers were to be trained as they needed information about mental illness - how to spot indications of the onset of instability, note the effects of medication and learn about the means of motivating patients in their care.

A club for residents had been established whose members met once a week. Apart from discussing issues pertaining to their own well-being, members visited those who were still in hospitals, and they joined in a number of activities in the community which facilitated their integration. Through the scheme, run by the Day Care Centre, some users were employed by local firms and COMCARE. Others did voluntary work in various institutions.

Funding Money for the establishment and the successful running of this organisation has come from a variety of sources.

Capital The first funding came from two families. As the organisation became a Trust more people donated. One day a man knocked at the door and handed a cheque for R200,000 to buy another house. Another way of raising funds was through families with financial means who wanted to invest in accommodation for their families. Using this method four families invested R100,000 each with which the Trust bought a block of 10 flats for independent living. In future the sons and daughters of these families will own these flats.

Running Costs It costs R1,200 a month to keep one person in a group home. Revenue for this came from rent and a government subsidy. Residents whose families could afford paid R750 a month. Those who had no supporting kinship systems paid R340 which was three quarters of their disability grant. The government subsidy was R281 a month for the first year and this was increased to R590 for subsequent years when there was proof that the money was well spent on the patient.

In concluding our interview the founder member of COMCARE made clear the relationship they have with hospitals:

> We started as a partnership between the community and the hospital. We do not question their professional expertise. We need them for medication. They need our support in the community. We both need each other. We monitor the effects of medication on patients and

housemothers have a list of side effects of different drugs. We monitor the effects of an increase or reduction of medication and relay that information to the professionals with whom we work closely.

In the task of supporting mentally ill people in the community and working closely with professionals in hospitals, COMCARE was working hand in hand with Fountain House, a local day care centre situated in the vicinity of many of the group homes.

Although COMCARE was established by white parents for their children who were diagnosed as schizophrenics, the organisation has opened its doors to all those who need its services. In 1995 a voluntary group in Mitchell's Plain, which was running a group home donated to them by a pharmaceutical company, approached COMCARE to take it over because it was not working effectively. Mitchell's Plain is a residential area predominantly used by the 'coloured' population. Unlike the private sector discussed above, finances are not a barrier. Even for those parents who must pay because they can afford it, R750 a month is nothing compared to R359 a day in the private sector. The strength of the organisation is in its commitment to re-integrate people back into their communities.

Fountain House

This was a Drop-in Centre for people with mental illness. The Centre worked closely with COMCARE and psychiatric hospitals in the area. It provided a variety of activities. Of particular interest was the involvement of members in employment. The Centre had developed links with different firms and organisations. Members were offered an opportunity to take part in the employment scheme. Those who were interested went through a preparatory stage in the Centre during which they had to prove that they had the necessary qualities required by employers, i.e. they must be punctual, reliable, well-groomed and willing to learn. When firms accepted employees from the Centre, staff had to guarantee that if a member was not able to go to work, for whatever reason, a member of staff would fill the gap. As the manager explained:

> We really have to work hard to convince employers to be part of this employment scheme. Even those who join it, they want a guarantee that their firms will not be disrupted by absenteeism from our members. That is why we have to take over when members do not turn up for work. The employers simply ring here, and one of us goes there to work.

Some members went back to their previous employment once they were discharged from hospital. The Centre formed links with the employers and that extended the support they gave to members.

Fountain House itself provided some employment. Some members were employed in the office as receptionists, editors of the newsletter or administrators compiling and maintaining a database. When I visited the Centre I was taken around by one of the receptionists who introduced me to staff and members in the Centre. Other members served in a shop which sold second-hand clothes, whilst others were responsible for the sale of candles and other artefacts made by members. The proceeds from all these sales went towards the members' fund which was managed by a treasurer.

The variety of activities offered in the Centre were important but the employment component had a central role in people's rehabilitation. It was the hope of all those who worked in this area, that the government would act on this knowledge in the re-organisation of the mental health services.

The Department of Health was in the process of re-organising mental health services. There were doubts about the extent to which services would be improved by this re-organisation. The COMCARE Committee believed that the government was not giving as much attention to mental health as it was to the rest of the health service. That had to change if effective care was to be made available to the growing number of mentally ill people, many of whom were young victims afflicted by the stresses of political violence. As the British experience has shown, community care must not be adopted to save money. It must be pursued with the genuine desire to link and integrate people in their communities. If that is to be achieved the input of the communities through the collaboration of NGOs is going to be crucial. That is why it is critical that relationship between NGOs and the government are healthy and co-operative.

References

Mental Health and Substance Abuse Committee (1996), Human Rights Violations and Alleged Malpractices in Psychiatric Institutions Report.

Seedat, A. (1984), *Crippling A Nation: Health in Apartheid South Africa*, International Defence and AID Fund for Southern Africa.

9 HIV/AIDS Epidemic

It is estimated that since the human immunodeficiency virus (HIV) made its appearance 30 million people have contracted the virus and six million have died of acquired immune deficiency syndrome (AIDS). Ninety per cent of the infected population live in 'developing countries' (Wolfesohn *et al*, 1997). Approximately 86 percent of those in third world countries live in sub-Sahara Africa and in South and South East Asia. In 1995 about 500,000 children were born with HIV infection and 67 percent of them were in sub-Saharan Africa, 30 percent in South and South East Asia and 2-3 percent in Latin America and the Caribbean (UNAIDS and WHO 1996). Statistics for South Africa are based on the Annual National Antenatal HIV figures collected from a sample of public clinics. The results of the surveys showed that the total number of women affected by the virus increased from 7.6 percent in 1994 to 14.1 percent in 1996. Extrapolation from these findings suggested that by 1996 1.4 million adults would be HIV positive (Floyd, 1997). The estimate for 1997 was that there would be about 90,000 new AIDS cases in South Africa and that 20,000 of those would be amongst children born to HIV infected mothers (Doyle and Muhr, 1996). In the 1998 survey 22.6 percent of pregnant women were HIV positive.

One of the questions that has been asked in relation to the extent of infection in 'developing' countries is why there is such a high rate when in fact regardless of race or class every person exposed to the virus can get AIDS. Sabatier gives a fairly comprehensive answer to the question:

> Once the AIDS (Acquired Immune Deficiency Syndrome) virus has entered a society, it tends towards the path of least resistance. Internationally, that line runs directly through some of the world's least powerful communities: the poorest, most disadvantaged groups whose members constitute an increasing disproportionate share of the world's total AIDS case. This includes communities of 'The Third World' decent, within some developed nations. AIDS is in reality the latest trend to emerge beside all those other epidemics - of infant mortality and malnutrition, of sexually transmitted and other diseases, of alcohol and

drug misuse and of psychological distress and social disruption - which disproportionately affect the disadvantaged.

The AIDS pandemic cannot be properly understood apart from this background, and it is arguable that AIDS will never be controlled, let alone eliminated, without a change in the combined conditions of underdevelopment, unbalanced development and political marginalisation which provide it with fertile soil (Sabatier, 1988).

The apartheid system in South Africa provided a very fertile path for the spread of AIDS, not only through the creation of poverty but also through its labour migratory system which left men in single sex hostel accommodation where some turned to each other for friendship and sexual intimacy. Students who conducted research in the mines reported that homosexual practices were seen as normal and were accepted by the inmates of the hostels (University Students, 1976). The consequence for the wives at home was that some men became accustomed to homosexual methods of having sex and they expected their wives to accept these practices in their conjugal relationship. The Observer reported the stress this caused for women when their husbands came home:

> ...and when he comes home I am frightened. He does strange things to me. I can't talk about these things, but other women say the same. It's because in the mines all they have for company is men. Sometimes I wish he would not come back, and just send me money. (Observer, 1978).

Little has changed since the ANC government has come to power. The migrant labour system still exists and it is no coincidence that AIDS is highest in those areas where the migrant labour system is dominant, e.g. KwaZulu-Natal 750,000, Gauteng 466,000 and Northern Cape 22,000 people affected (Floyd, 1997).

Another product of the apartheid system is the de-valuing of black people's lives, not only at the macro level but also at a micro level in the delivery of health services. When administering an injection it was not an unusual practice for some GPs to use the same syringe and needle for more than one patient. One woman told of her reaction to this practice:

> A number of us were sitting there waiting to be treated. The dentist came with a 10cc syringe full of local anaesthetic. He moved from one person to the next, injecting them with small amounts of the fluid without even changing the needle. When I saw that I just took my bag and left.

The factors mentioned are not solely responsible for the rapid spread of AIDS in South Africa but they do need to be taken into consideration when explanations are sought for the escalation of AIDS. The education needed is not just for the users but also for the health professionals and government officers, to ensure that these factors are dealt with alongside other measures aimed at minimising the risk of infection.

Managing HIV/AIDS

By 1992 there were already signs that the HIV infection was on the increase. The Nationalist Government convened The National AIDS Convention of South Africa (NACOSA), with a mandate to develop a national AIDS strategy with technical assistance from WHO (Floyd, 1997). The NACOSA plan had six components:

- education and prevention;
- counselling;
- health care;
- human rights and law reform;
- welfare;
- research.

These components underpinned the management of HIV/AIDS and are still used by the ANC government to fight the virus albeit in ways that have sometimes earned it criticism. One of the criticisms was around the 'Virodene' cure claim made by a group of scientists at the University of Pretoria. The concern was about the response of the government to the claim:

> While the claims were soon debunked, and the 'cure' exposed as no more than an industrial solvent, questions lingered over why the health ministry had invited these three 'unknowns' in the AIDS field to present their work to Cabinet and to request R3.7 million in state funding when established scientists, who had been working on AIDS for many years with little funding, received no such breaks (Barron et al, 1997).

Treatment for AIDS

In Western Europe and North America the phrase 'post-AIDS' is becoming a familiar one for those who are involved in treating patients with the new combination therapies which include the use of protease inhibitors (Gatter, 1998).

This breakthrough has excited clinical researchers and practitioners who feel that now they can offer individualised patient management which will prolong good quality life. This excitement is captured in the Lancet:

> Recent developments have greatly altered the management of HIV-infected patients and we can expect further expansion in the range of treatment regimens and the arrival of new and more sensitive laboratory tools, such as plasma viral load assays, that permit greater individualisation of patient management (British HIV Association, 1997).

This is indeed a wonderful breakthrough for both medicine and patients who benefit from the new drugs. A patient in England who is on this treatment captured the magic effect of the treatment:

> I was very reluctant to go on this treatment because I was afraid of possible side effects, but I was also taking alternative therapy which I believed was going to help me. My condition got worse, I lost weight and I was very, very ill. The doctors told me that unless I went on this treatment I would die. I accepted I was going to die but then I thought of my family and decided to take the treatment. It worked very quickly for me, within 3 days I knew I was improving. I knew I was getting better because the white stuff on my tongue started to disappear.

At the time of the interview this patient looked healthy, energetic and was full of plans for the future. Despite these obvious successes however, some people remain concerned about the overall impact these drugs will have in the field of HIV/AIDS. Gatter maintains that if HIV/AIDS is no longer seen as implying permanent disablement, then funding for prevention and care services, and the balance between them will change:

> Care budgets are shifting towards supplying expensive drugs within primary rather than secondary care. Specialist HIV services providing social and residential care, particularly those in the Voluntary Sector, face severe budget cuts. The emphasis in prevention is moving towards

greater encouragement of HIV – antibody testing (for example, Crusaid's recent 'infovert') campaign (Gatter, 1998, p.10).

Gatter argues that changes will also have profound effects on people who have lived with HIV for a long time. Relative recovery of good health may attract pressure for people to return to work after years of unemployment. It is hard enough for unemployed people without HIV to get jobs. If they did get a job, would it pay enough to maintain the standard of living provided by the Disability Living Allowance?:

> To maintain a comparable standard of living someone who has been receiving, say, the maximum Disability Living Allowance would have to find a job with an annual salary approaching £20,000 a year. And after years out of employment, an individual may well be an unattractive prospect for employers (Gatter, p.10).

Jobs paying that level of salary are rare even for people without the AIDS virus. It can be assumed that some of the HIV infected people would not be able to get such jobs and a reduction in their standard of living would have a negative effect on their health status.

The other concern about these medical breakthroughs is that they are new and their long-term effect is not yet known:

> It is possible that someone may return to work and later become ill again, only to find that most of the health and social benefits, together with the impressive facilities set up in the late 1980s and early 1990s have vanished (Gatter, p.10).

In the world's desperation to find a cure these concerns can be dismissed. However, in the light of Alcorn's assertion Gatter's fears begin to make sense:

> ... there is growing evidence that some people with HIV are being denied powerful new treatments purely on the grounds of cost (Alcorn, 1996).

It costs £2,000 per year to treat one patient with AZT monotherapy and it is estimated that the new three combination drugs of, AZT, 3TC and Indinavir cost £7,000 per year. If the cost is prohibitive for the affluent Western countries what hope has South Africa of accessing these drugs? As in most cases, the cost will eventually come down and the drugs will be available to all those who need them. But can South Africa, or indeed any country, afford to wait for that time to arrive when it buries its young on a daily basis? The 'Virodene' incidence is an indication of the intensity in the search for an AIDS cure even among the 'unknowns'.

In its vision for the National Health Service encapsulated in the 1994 RDP, the government called for the elimination of divisions between those groups which provide health services. In particular it called for improved communication and co-operation between different types of healers in the interest of people who use them. Over 80 percent of black people use the services of traditional healers. It is to be expected therefore that when people suffer from AIDS they will consult traditional healers as part of their own search for a cure. The government is aware of this and so are some of the health workers who are involved in providing health care at an operational level. Whilst some of these health personnel dismiss traditional healing as 'mumbojumbo', others are not as hasty to write it off in this way because they have witnessed some improvement in people's conditions after being treated with traditional medicine.

A nurse working in the Admissions Unit explained why she does not dismiss traditional healing:

> People in our hospital are diagnosed as having AIDS. They are admitted and treated. After some time they are discharged because doctors have decided there is nothing more they can do and the patient is expected to die. After discharge some people go to traditional healers for treatment and they recover. When they come to hospital with other illnesses we check them for HIV. The results for many of them are negative. There is a young woman who had meningitis. She could not sit up without being supported. She was discharged to die at home. She was treated with traditional medicine and she recovered. She is very healthy at the moment. She continues to take the mixture. Another young girl, who was diagnosed in 1992, had lost weight and had diarrhoea. She too went to traditional healers and she is still fine.

The same informant also reported that the observed remission is temporary since some of the patients come back in a terminal state:

> We admit at least three or four patients a day who have been treated by traditional healers. It looks as if they get better from taking the mixture and they can be free from symptoms for a long time, some for two or three years but when they stop treatment the disease suddenly comes back and is more aggressive. They die within months of falling ill again.

It is difficult to conclude from this information whether or not the observed improvement is the result of African medicine since little research has been done in this area. What is interesting, however, is that a similar aggressive relapse occurs when treatment with the three-combination drug is discontinued. The patient on the combination drugs knew of other patients who had had such relapses:

> One girl who stopped taking the medication died within months. Another one who stopped when on holiday is now extremely ill in hospital. But the thing is if you miss taking the treatment at the times you are supposed to, then it won't work anymore. The HIV mutates and people have to be moved to another combination. Some people stop just for a weekend and the virus becomes resistant. You see, there is a limit to the combinations to which people can be moved. The thing is you have to keep the levels up in your body, if they fall as they do when you stop taking the treatment even for a short time the virus mutates and becomes very aggressive. I feel so good, I will never stop taking the treatment. The only thing is, will it always be available? They tell us that it is very expensive and that some health authorities can only have so many patients.

Is there a common factor in the two forms of treatment? This question cannot be answered until the arena in the search for a cure is opened up to the 'unknowns' including traditional healers whose activities impact on the lives of a high proportion of black people. Whatever perception health workers have of traditional healers, communication and co-operation in the interest of the users must be established. As the President of the South African Traditional Healers Association observed, South African doctors are still not keen to establish this relationship:

> People come from all over the world to see what I do and how I work but South African medical doctors don't come, so they don't know whether we kill our patients or what we do (Ewing 1998, p.16).

If there is ambiguity about the role of traditional healers in the cure of AIDS, there is no such doubt about the role they play in managing people with AIDS:

> ... one of the main reasons that traditional healers remain so popular and trusted (aside from affordability and accessibility) is because they focus on the well-being of the patient, not simply the treatment of his or her condition (Ewing, p.17).

References

Alcorn, K. (1996), 'The Cost of Treatment', *AIDS Treatment Update*, November, issue 47.

Barron, P., Strachan, K. and Ijsselmuiden, C. (1997), 'The Year in Review', *Health Systems Trust*.

British HIV Association (1997), 'Guidelines for antiretroviral treatment of HIV seropositive individuals', *The Lancet*, vol.349, No.958, pp.1086-1092.

Doyle, P. and Muhr, T. (1996), *Seventh National HIV Survey of Women attending antenatal clinics of the public health services*, October/November.

Ewing, D. (1998), 'Traditional Healing – Back to our Roots', *Children First*, vol.2, No.16.

Floyd, E. (1997), 'HIV/AIDS', *South African Health Review*, Health Systems Trust, pp.187-197.

Gatter, P. (1998), 'HIV & AIDS', *Research Matters*, April-October.

Sabatier, R. (1988), *Blaming Others: Prejudice, Race and Worldwide AIDS*, The Panos Institute.

The Observer Magazine, 11 June 1978.

UNIADS and WHO, (1996), 'The HIV/AIDS situation in mid 1996 Global and Regional Highlights', *Fact Sheet 1*, July.

University Students (1976), *Another Blanket*, Agency Industry Mission.

Wolfensohn, J.D., de Beus P. and Joào Piot, P. (1997), *Confronting AIDS, Public Priorities in a Global Epidemic*, The World Bank.

10 Care for Terminally Ill People – The Role of Hospices

Although my research interest has always been on health, care for terminally ill people has never been the focus of attention. I suspect that one of the reasons for this omission is that in my conventional concept of health, inherited from my previous training, death and care for the dying did not feature high. Even in the present research my initial contact with the people who provide care for terminally ill people in South Africa was purely accidental rather than by design.

In Cape Town I happened to live in a house which was situated opposite St Luke's Hospice. Joan, in whose house I lived, took in exchange nurses from England who worked in the Centre. Even though none of them were in the house when I was there, hospice work formed part of our general conversation on health matters and it was in that context that my research interest in the care of terminally ill people was developed.

Through Joan I managed to get access to the hospice and its staff.

St Luke's Hospice

Information on the history and activities of St. Luke's Hospice was collected from interviews with members of staff in the education, community development and nursing sectors of the organisation. The hospice dates back to 1979 when Dame Cicely, initiator of the hospice movement visited Cape Town. Her inspiration led to a series of seminars and discussions by concerned people which led to the establishment of the hospice in 1980. The aim was to care for all terminally ill people in need of its services regardless of their ability to pay. After moving sites the organisation finally found suitable premises in Kenilworth in 1989.

St. Luke's is one of the 45 hospices in South Africa and one of six in the Western Cape. The number of terminally ill people who used the Centre was 15,000. Referrals were from doctors/hospitals, social workers, clinics and families.

Between 1989 and 1992 the Board of Directors decided to introduce the hospice concept into the community. Communities were encouraged to set up their own hospices which became satellites of St. Luke's.

To support the newly formed satellite St Luke's provided a trained nursing sister with a car to look after 25 patients in their own homes. If more people needed the service then the committee had to find extra funding. The satellites negotiated their own constitution but they had to abide by the ethos of the mother organisation.

The community development officer whose function was to encourage the concept of hospice in the community explained that fund raising in the black community was not easy because of people's economic status. This made it difficult to rent premises for day-care services and in consequence patients were admitted in the main centre for symptom control and respite for carers.

After referral patients were allocated to nursing sisters who worked closely with all the people who interacted with the patient. These included family, friends, social workers, doctors and teachers if there were children of school age. In every activity undertaken the patient remained the central agent. The patient was offered what was available and she/he decided whether or not what was offered was acceptable. The main function of the sister was to work out options for patients as they visited them in their homes. One of the nursing sisters invited me to accompany her on her home visits.

Home Visits

We visited a number of families with terminally ill patients. I was very moved by the ease with which she talked about the imminent death with the patient and family members. She spent her time with each family as if that was her only job. She never made them feel that she had another patient to see. She encouraged her patients and their families to discuss any issue that was worrying them. It was time for them to tell their dying relative whatever was worrying them about the relationship they have had with them. But it was not only the negative that had to be cleared but the positive as well. 'Tell your mother how much you love her', she told one young woman'. Let her know how much you have appreciated all that she has meant to you. Don't worry about the fact that she does not respond. I can assure you she hears everything you say'. In addition to this pastoral role the sister administered a variety of treatments needed by her patients.

On our way back I commented on the difference between the patients we had seen. I was particularly struck by the calm and the peacefulness of two of the patients we had visited. She introduced me to all her patients. One woman was very interested when she heard that I was a visitor from England. She asked me to sit next to her and she held my hand. She asked questions about England as if it actually mattered to her even though she knew she had less that a couple of days to live. She asked if I had any family. She created such a tranquil atmosphere that I told her about deaths in my family as if it was the most normal everyday thing to happen in every family. We were so relaxed about death that when I was leaving and we were still holding hands I said to her, 'now when you get to the pearly gates, if my two who have gone there do not put the red carpet out when you arrive, tell them that they will have to answer to me when I get there'. She laughed and said, 'I hope they will also have prepared a curry dinner. I have not had that for months. What are their names?' I told her, and she said, 'I will remember them', and gently squeezing my hand said, 'and I will not forget their mother. Go back well to England. We will meet again'.

The next patient we visited was the direct opposite. She was very restless and in pain. She hardly said anything unless it was to complain about something. She tossed and turned in her bed. She barely heard the sister when she introduced me. When we arrived in the house there was nobody with her. The acquaintance who looked after her whilst the family was at work came in soon after we arrived. The sister gave the patient a suppository to relieve the pain and had a talk to her about the possibility of coming in for a few days to the Centre for rest and the control of pain. We left with the sister promising to call again later in the day.

Our third visit was to a patient who was as peaceful as the first one except she hardly communicated with anyone. The sister introduced me. She opened her eyes and looked at me. When we left she put her hand out and held mine and whispered, 'God bless you'. In this house the sister spent most of her time talking to the daughter who was very upset about the mother's condition and about things that she felt she needed to tell her before she died.

The sister explained the difference between her patients in terms of their state of mind as a result of what she called 'unfinished matters' in the family. In the family of the restless woman there was a lot of conflict between the mother and her children, a conflict that went back for years. The sister had been working with the family in an attempt to resolve these conflicts. The sister only gets involved if she is invited to do so by the patient.

Comments

To some people it may appear inappropriate to spend time looking at the work of the hospice in a research in which the aim is to look at the health needs of people and the ways in which they might be improved. But in actual fact the work of the hospice is doing precisely that. It is allowing people to have a healthy death and to that extent its work fits in well with a comprehensive definition of health. In death, just as in health, there are glaring inequalities. Another family we visited was in an informal settlement. The patient who suffered from cancer had asked to be taken into the main Centre for a break from the intolerable conditions in her home. I saw their home when the sister was taking the father and the children back after they had been to see the mother. The settlement was in the middle of nowhere, totally surrounded by a forest. There were 40 families, all living in small shacks made of cardboard and bits and pieces of planks and plastic. They were so close to each other that if one caught fire the others would be burnt down as well. They showed us a site where one shack was burnt down the week before and by sheer luck people woke up in time to prevent the fire spreading, but not in time to save the owner of the shack who was burnt to death. There were no toilets, people used the forest and as a result there was a toilet smell surrounding the settlement and flies had access to both forest and people's dwellings. The house we were visiting had three beds which practically filled the whole area except for a small space for a two burner paraffin stove and some pots and pans. That was the entire living space for a family of five. It was difficult to visualise what kind of life the family led when they were all well, let alone when one of them was dying of cancer. The husband was unemployed. I asked the sister what the role of the hospice was in those situations where the patient may not even have enough food to eat:

> Well, the work of the hospice is not about the social needs but about death. So we do not provide food or beds. We have no capacity to do that. But we work very closely with social workers who respond to the needs of our patients as far as it is possible.

My involvement with the work of St. Luke's Hospice encouraged me to visit Houghton Hospice in Gauteng Province.

Houghton Hospice

The establishment of this hospice was also motivated by a talk by Dame Cicely in 1979. The property on which the present Centre is based was acquired in 1984 with donations from various sources. The mission, ethos and philosophy are the same as those that guide the operations in St Luke's. It is a smaller organisation with a capacity for 18 in-patient beds with only 10 of them in occupancy because of financial constraints. The hospice operates on R4 million a year. The Centre is located in a white Johannesburg suburb, miles from the black community, with poor travelling facilities. We asked the Director how available was the service to black people:

> My rough estimate is that about 30 percent of patients who come here are black. But I think there are a lot more people who could use this service out there. The problem is that nobody really knows the extent of cancer in the country because statistics have not been kept after the apartheid regime was dismantled.

However, in recent years a number of factors have combined to put pressure on the hospice staff to think of ways in which the needs of black people can be met within their service. The expansion in primary health care, in particular the mobile clinic units means that more people with cancer will be identified. The rise in the number of people with AIDS has put pressure on terminal care services. To meet the need would Houghton emulate the satellite scheme?

> No, not really, not for us here. We have a very large population to cover. Soweto alone has over two million people. This place is not only inaccessible but it is also too small to cope with the need when more people begin to use the service. At the moment in Soweto there are two professional nurses who work in the community. They work from home and only come here once a week for supervision and meetings. We know that this is not enough but the St Luke's' model is not the answer (Houghton Director, 1997).

The answer was not in creating satellites but in building a Centre which would replicate facilities in Houghton. But it was not only the size of the black population in Soweto which militated against the Cape Town model. The Director pointed out that one needs to take into account the historical economic, political and social development of the country when making decisions about health provision:

> The idea of satellites raising their own funds is not acceptable for two main reasons. One is that there is unequal availability of resources between groups. There are rich areas, mainly white, which will be able to raise large sums of money for their communities, and poor areas, mainly black, which will be starved of resources. The net result would be an exclusive service in one area and a poor one in another. We need a cross subsidy in this country. It is for this reason that we think it is important to pool resources in order to distribute according to the needs of the individual centre. All the centres will have their own management structure and fund raising, but they will all be linked to the mother centre which will also raise funds, maintain the centres and pay salaries. But it is a collective responsibility based on cross fertilisation in fund raising. The other is that when funding is directed to autonomous satellites, the main centre will be starved of funds and will not be able to meet its own obligation of maintaining equity in service provision. For this reason we think it is important to pool resources in one main centre which then distributes according to the needs of individual centres (Houghton Director, 1997).

The intention was to build four centres in different townships which would link up with primary health care services. The managers of Houghton Hospice had already been invited by the Local Council of Orange Farm to discuss the possibility of providing training for the needs of the terminally ill people in the area. The initiative came from the community:

> We are listening to what the communities want. Our intention is to build these four centres. But of course this will be dependent on the ability to raise funds. But we are not inflexible. As things develop there may be changes, the system is open to new ideas (Director, 1997).

Both the Cape Town and the Johannesburg hospices concentrated on urban areas. Was there any service for communities in the rural areas? Portshepstone Hospice which focuses more on rural communities would be a good one to visit, the Director advised.

The Portshepstone Hospice

The service was set up in Portshepstone Hospital which was used by patients from rural areas who presented with cancer of the oesophagus and cervix. On discharge the patients were given a month's supply of liquid morphine and they were expected to come back for repeat prescriptions. However, many patients found it difficult to come back because of their weakened condition, as well as difficulty in transportation. As a result many patients stayed at home and did without any medication. It was for these reasons that the team started a rural outreach programme. The demand was so great that the staff could not manage without help. To ease the workload a link was made with Murchison, a rural hospital which had satellite clinics. The Co-founder of the hospice, now the Director of the Centre, remembers the first black patient they treated in Murchison hospital:

> His name was Elias and he was referred by a priest. This was in the early 1990s, a time of high political unrest and although Elias was in severe pain he would not accept us until we had given evidence that we were not working for the Nationalist Government. We told him that we were not working for the government but for God. He was our first patient and through him we were allowed to run a hospice service in Murchison based on pain control (Hospice Director, 1997).

In time the team was able to train some of the staff members in the hospital in caring for terminally ill patients. The work went beyond hospital boundaries as staff became voluntary carers in their neighbourhoods. The network worked very well until it was disrupted by intense political violence which endangered the lives of nurses:

> A home of one of the staff members was burnt down endangering not just her life but also that of her whole family. This was because she went to treat a terminally ill patient after work. She was deemed to be supporting the opposing political party to which the patient belonged (Hospice Director, 1997).

Hospice work in the community was not, however, brought to a total halt by the political violence. A small flame remained which was later rekindled in the partnership between the hospice and comprehensive primary health care teams. The aim was to have in each of the clinics a nurse who was skilled in palliative care. The nurses do a six month day release course in Durban with Portshepstone Hospice providing a placement for practical skills. The course is approved by the South African Nursing Council which gives a certificate to successful students. As a result of this partnership, hospice work has been taken deep into rural areas.

In the township the Centre has made links with clinic staff who are willing to work as volunteers in their neighbourhoods. They visit the sick and give them basic nursing care in their own homes. One of the nurses serves as a co-ordinator and draws a list of people available at different times. She is also a link for other community groups that want to use the services of the hospice. One such group is a circle of church people who have a commitment to pastoral care for their members. Within the group are health professionals employed in different sectors of the health service. During the research in the KwaZulu-Natal province I stayed with one of these professionals which enabled me to accompany them when they were doing their community voluntary health care.

The patient was a middle-aged woman who lived with her grown up children. She was in the last stages of cancer of the uterus. Most of her bodily functions were failing. She had an impacted rectum which needed clearing manually. She had a catheter *in situ* but the tube leading to the bag was blocked and the heavily concentrated urine was flowing back giving her immense pain. The volunteer nurses checked her and concluded that this had created some infection and that the catheter needed changing. They discussed with the patient and the family the possibility of going to the hospice centre for pain control and relief of symptoms. This visit was late in the evening but since the clinic based co-ordinator of the group was on night duty, she was informed about the condition and what needed to be done and she made all the necessary arrangements. The following day the patient was transferred to the hospice centre in town.

A few days later a phone call came from one of the children to say that the mother was dying. The members of the church team who were off work arranged to take the family and friends to the bedside of the patient. Most of the time was spent praying and talking to the patient who was calm and comfortable with no pain at all. We left her with her daughter who promised to keep the team informed. The patient died peacefully four weeks after this visit and in that time the team members who worked near the hospice visited her regularly.

The increase in the number of people suffering from AIDS has put a lot of pressure on hospice work and to cope with the demand, partnerships are being established with central government funding bodies. In the spirit of this co-operation the Portshepstone Hospice, in partnership with Murchison Hospital, the Primary Health-Care network and the HIV/AIDS Regional team was given the sum of R250,000 for an AIDS programme. The project employed two community workers who were trained to nurse patients as well as teach families how to nurse their own relatives and how to protect themselves from infection. The workers were monitored on a daily basis by the project supervisor, a professional nurse, based at Murchison Hospital. The whole focus of the project was on home-care with back-up by means of emergency beds, rural Primary Health Care clinics and the hospice which provided overall co-ordination, training and equipment.

The elimination of inequalities at death is as important as the elimination of inequalities in health. Dying with human dignity should not be determined by race, class or gender. By taking the concept of hospice to the black community the above organisations are taking a necessary step. Each organisation is following a different path to achieve the same objective, an inclusive care system for all needing terminal care. The paths, as the directors of these organisations pointed out, are informed by the circumstances in their individual areas. This granted, there is no reason why a combination of approaches cannot be adopted in one geographical area in order to reach as many people as possible.

Acknowledging the reservation about autonomous fund raising, it is quite feasible, for example, for the township centres that Houghton hopes to develop, to have hospice stations in clinics and other community centres as well as in doctors' surgeries to ensure that people do not travel for miles to get to the main centre. There is also no reason why St Luke's and Houghton hospices cannot follow the path taken by the Portshepstone Hospice in reaching out to communities in rural areas. The major problem faced by all these organisations is funding and it is here that partnerships with the government must be encouraged, not just for AIDS patients but for all terminally ill patients.

11 The Orange Farm Study

Orange Farm is recognised as one of the biggest informal settlements in South Africa. Statistics from the latest census indicate that there are just under one million people living in the area, but those who work and live there believe that this is an underestimation. To facilitate geographical location the area is divided into numbered sections called extensions. Another division is based on the kind of houses in which people live. There is the older part with brick built houses, very much like the old four-roomed style of the traditional township homes. The other part of Orange Farm is composed of imikhukhu (shacks), made of anything that people can find - corrugated iron sheets, cardboard and plastic sheets. Although some of these structures are of reasonable size, the majority are very small reflecting the families' economic ability to find building materials.

The Origins of Orange Farm

Under the apartheid regime the residency status of people was governed by law which divided people into groups A, B, C and D. Under A were all residents born in the township. B was allocated to men who moved into the area. Women who moved into the township were given a C status even if they were married to men in the B category. Farm labourers were given a D status. Only group A people had full entitlement to all facilities available in the city within which the township was located – employment, education, health services, housing, business licences etc. Men in the B category attained the same entitlement after ten years, but women and farm labourers did not qualify for services irrespective of the length of residency. The existing townships therefore were not very welcoming places for people who came to Johannesburg from rural areas in search of a better life. Besides these residency restrictions, townships like Soweto were themselves experiencing intense overcrowding as the numbers of those born in the township increased.

The opportunity to escape the pressure that many people were experiencing was offered by a white farmer who decided to change the use of his farm. Farmer Weiler owned a farm not far from Soweto. He had a large number of farm workers for whom he provided houses. In 1981 Weiler decided to stop farming. Apart from the fact that he was getting on in years, he also had the delusion that there were masses and masses of gold in his farm and in order to access it he employed people to dig for it. He rented out the houses formerly used by his farm workers as well as renting out plots of land to people who wanted to build their own shacks. The place was flooded by farm workers who had been thrown out of white farms, people who had low residency status in the existing townships, township-born people escaping high rents and overcrowding as well as people from rural areas in search of a better life in the city. The rents were R20 a month. One informant who rented a farm worker's house described the mood of the people at the time:

> We had to pay farmer Weiler R20 a month. At first people paid but later they did not. I never paid. I saw no reason to. This was our land and all we wanted was to have a place to live. It was there, empty, and I saw no reason why I should pay for it (ex resident, 1997).

Unlike some white farmers who provided schools for their labourer's children, farmer Weiler did not:

> He wanted children to be farm workers like their parents and felt that education might give them ideas above their station (ex resident).

That was why when the new settlers came there was no school for their children. The newcomers formed a resident's committee which decided to set up a school. A member of the group offered her house to be used for classrooms:

> In 1985 we started from sub A to standard six. That gave the children eight years of education. Sub A was the biggest class, so we had them in the kitchen which was the biggest room in the house. Other classes were held in the bedrooms and under the trees. We had no facilities. We used to go to factories and beg for large sheets of paper which we hung on trees and used as writing boards. We collected dishes in which supermarkets sold meat and used them as teaching aids. We drew apples, animals, words and figures on them (ex resident, 1997).

The committee found financial and moral support from the South African Council of Churches and, locally, had the full support of Bishop Desmond Tutu. In 1986 class seven was added and in 1988 class eight was established. By this time a number of organisations were already supporting the school financially. The Royal Netherlands was paying for teachers' salaries, the Gatehead Foundation was donating money and the Australian Embassy was providing furniture. Farmer Weiler was not very happy with what was happening on his farm. On a number of occasions he called in the police to arrest a tenant not only for using her house as a school but also for teaching illegally, as he saw it. The police did arrest her and she was bailed for R1000. The women responded with a subtle non-confrontational protest. One woman who took part in this protest remembered how angry but impotent the prison officials were:

> We deliberately collected R1 coins and filled buckets which we carried on our heads and went to prison singing our protest songs. We watched them count every coin. They were angry but they could do nothing about it (ex resident, 1997).

One of the reasons why the authorities felt impotent was that the Black Sash, a white women's organisation which was very active in fighting apartheid, was providing legal aid and guidance for the running of the school. They knew therefore that any harassment of the women would not only be the subject of media coverage but would also be raised in Parliament since some of the Sash women were members of the Progressive Party. In addition, in legal terms, the women had committed no crime even under the apartheid regime.

The addition of standard eight, which had to be certificated officially, presented problems for the school because as far as the main stream education system was concerned, it did not exist since it was not registered. A Roman Catholic school for white pupils in Yoeville came to the rescue in the person of Brother Neil who provided books and teachers to raise the academic level of the pupils. He then enrolled them under his school so that they could sit mainstream examinations. By 1986 the government realising that Weiler had no intention to farm his land, expropriated it, declared it a transit camp, and used it to accommodate the soldiers and police. Their pastime was intimidating and harassing the residents:

> They were really horrible. When people came back from shopping, they took their food and ate it. They took people's cars and drove them around and broke them. One time they undressed a man and forced him to go naked all the way to his house. They used to collect youngsters in their jeeps, take them up to the mountain and beat them up, breaking their teeth in the process. The Indian community used to come to the settlement to

feed the children. On one occasion the soldiers came whilst the children were eating and spread tear gas in the room (ex resident, 1997).

The committee decided enough was enough and called on all the residents to challenge the perpetrators. They phoned the Black Sash to tell them what they intended doing. Helen Suzman, a member of the Progressive Party, informed the relevant Minister who instructed the chief of police to fly out in a helicopter and negotiate with the chairperson and ask her to talk to the residents:

> I talked to the residents and we agreed to disband and talk to the chief of police. But we had had enough of the harassment. You see, we were in a white area and white residents did not want us there. They too were pushing the local authority to harass us. They put pressure on their local councillors. We had no vote and nobody to speak on our behalf. Even when the soldiers and police abused us, nobody was prepared to defend us. People were killed and the authorities did nothing about it. Strydom, the police officer who shot over ten black people during lunch time in Pretoria, passed through Weiler's farm and tested the efficiency of his gun by shooting at the shacks. Two young girls were shot dead in their sleep and nothing was done about it by the authorities (Chair, 1997).

It was not only systematic harassment that motivated the residents of Weiler's farm to move out of the area. There was still no secure education for their children. They still relied on other people's goodwill for both funding and certification. They did not own the land on which they built their shacks. They still could not have licences if they wanted to open a business. It was for these reasons that when the Government expropriated a number of farms in the area now known as Orange Farm, the residents of Weiler's farm were eager to go, even though they knew that this was being established as a dumping ground for black people.

The first families moved into Orange Farm in October 1988. Each family was given the opportunity to purchase a site which was 11 by 20 meters for R500. For the first time people owned their own piece of land. The government, eager to see people move into Orange Farm, facilitated a house building scheme through the National Housing Commission which was administered by the Transvaal Provincial Administration (TPA).

The idea was for the TPA to build houses which would then be sold for R8,000. People were to pay monthly instalments and the money collected would be used to build more houses. The idea was good but it did not benefit the people who came from Weiler's farm:

Firstly, the TPA officials got together with white contractors and took the money for their own use. Some contractors were paid without finishing the building which meant that many people had to finish the work on their own homes. As a result people refused to pay the monthly instalments and this in turn slowed down the house building programme. Secondly, people from Weiler's farm wanted black contractors to build their homes but the white officials processing the forms, did not send those from black contractors to Pretoria which meant that they could not be paid. The exclusion of black contractors from the system meant that many of us were left with no houses and we remained in the shacks for a very long time until we could build our own homes. The only people who really benefited from the scheme were those who chose white contractors to build their homes (ex resident, 1997).

Why Orange Farm for a Localised Study?

A combination of factors made Orange Farm appropriate for a localised study of health needs. The first was its location. Unlike the other informal settlements which are attached to or are near existing townships, Orange Farm is in the middle of nowhere. It lies between Gauteng (Johannesburg) and Verenniging. There are hardly any services in the form of retailing facilities. For groceries people rely on tuck shops which operate in people's homes, in shacks or open stalls in different locations which have gained themselves the status of 'market' place. There are obvious health implications when food is sold in this way. In the 'market' place it was not unusual to see defrosted chicken pieces, exposed to the sun and dust from passing vehicles, still being sold in the afternoon. Apart from the health hazard, there is also a diminution in nutritional content when fruit and vegetables are left exposed to the heat of the sun. This is particularly the case with Vitamin C. Even if people were balancing their diet, they would not only miss out on some nutrients but would also be in danger of food-poisoning.

The second factor was the size of the settlement and the consequent numbers of people affected by the socio-economic status of the area, and the impact of that status on health. The third factor was meeting people who lived or worked in Orange Farm who were keen to bring about positive changes in order to benefit people in the area.

Methodology

In undertaking this study a combination of methods were employed. It was through 'living with people' that I was introduced to Orange Farm. During a lunch break at a Women's Conference we exchanged information about the areas in which we were involved. A woman in the group who heard that I was particularly interested in looking at health needs in rural and peri-urban communities gave me contact names for Orange Farm. It was through following this lead that I made contact with the Women's Voice of Orange Farm. On a separate occasion I was given the name of a general practitioner whose surgery provided health services to some of the people who live in Orange Farm. These contacts introduced me to other relevant people, and through this snowballing process a series of in-depth interviews were carried out. Information collected in these interviews was later supported, clarified and verified when I visited projects mentioned by interviewees. In addition to individual interviews, group discussions were held during which community members raised concerns about health and health-related issues. It was from these in-depth interviews and group discussions that the health needs of Orange Farm were identified.

Facilities in Orange Farm

The first people to move into Orange Farm had hardly any facilities. They built their homes with whatever they could find just as they did on Weiler's farm. They had to dig their own pit latrines. There was one water tap available for every 415 families. There were no shops for daily needs and no schools. There were no job opportunities and those who found employment in the cities had to contend with expensive and poor transport facilities. There were hardly any health facilities. It was, as one informant stressed, 'a real dumping ground'. Gradually the situation changed. Some people moved into houses. Tuck shops for daily needs sprang up in homes and in 'market' places. Schools were built and some doctors moved into the area. These changes served the early arrivals. In the meantime a large number of people arrived and built more shacks for their homes. They came from different sources - farm workers thrown out of white farms; people from rural areas escaping political violence; those in search of a better life in the cities and those escaping from crowded township family homes.

In the 1990s the political climate began to change visibly. Orange Farm was supplied with electricity. In 1996 a sewerage system was introduced in some parts of the informal settlement. However, newcomers to the area had still to dig their own pit latrines, and in a crowded place like Orange Farm, this created serious health problems.

Health facilities leave a lot to be desired. There are only five doctors and four clinics serving a population estimated to be nearer two million by some people who live there. I visited one clinic in the shack area. The area is so vast that people at the margins have to walk a long distance to get to the clinic. Like many other clinics that I visited, this was crowded with very few staff to cope with the workload. Community-trained registered nurses diagnosed and treated patients and local GPs provided sessional consultations.

Although the residents of Orange Farm are not tenants anymore, there are still restrictions on what they can do with the land on which their homes are built. This is because of the law which governs the expropriation of land in South Africa. Some land has mineral rights which belong to the original owners or their relatives. If the owners cannot be traced in five years their land rights are forfeited. Until the issue of ownership rights is settled the residents of Orange Farm could not have the deeds to their homes, could not have a bond (mortgage) for building a house or establishing a business. The resolution of the proclamation question was delayed by events that overtook the country. These included the release of President Mandela and other political prisoners, the 1994 General Elections, the 1995 local elections and the deployment process. As a result Orange Farm was left with hardly any meaningful business ventures for many years.

Community Health Needs

One of the people I met in Orange Farm was a G.P. who I shall call Dr Nta who has a surgery adjacent to Orange Farm. Many of the patients who use the surgery come from Orange Farm. Dr. Nta had a very holistic view of health. He spent a lot of time taking me around different townships and informal settlements, pointing out the social and economic conditions under which people lived. After rain many roads remained submerged under water because of poor drainage. Football pitches were covered with water and on many occasions houses were flooded. In some areas household refuse littered the streets and was dumped in heaps near where children played. The Council was refusing to provide services because some people were not paying rent. The residents' argument was that the houses were badly built with cracks and other defects and they blamed the

Council for this because they felt that it was siding with the contractors instead of taking them to task for the shoddy work.

One area of concern for Dr. Nta was the welfare of children. He was a member of a committee which was running a crèche. Sixty seven children were packed into two rooms each measuring about 9 x 6 metres. The fee was R50 a month but since most parents could not afford to pay the whole amount the Committee had to raise funds for food and rent. At the time of the research, the committee was also raising funds to establish a purpose-built crèche which would have enough space for a garden to grow fresh food for the children.

It was also this commitment to the welfare of children that motivated Dr. Nta to lead a campaign for a safe road crossing for children:

> Taxis and private cars used to race through this road which is used by children going to school. There were no pedestrian crossings, no traffic lights and no speed checking devices. We told the council to do something about this but they paid no attention until a small girl was knocked down and killed by a car when she was crossing the road. We started a campaign on road safety. The community got together, marched with the children and forced the council to respond. Now the road has 'sleeping policemen' and that has slowed the cars down. We also encouraged local schools to start safety training for the children (Dr. Nta, 1997).

Dr. Nta was also aware of the political tension which divided the youth in the area. This was reflected in the use of the local stadium. If one group used it the other would not. Dr. Nta, who was well known and respected by both sides through his involvement with young people in the AIDS campaign, was trying various ways of bringing the youth together through sport.

It was during these visits with Dr. Nta to various sites that I saw the conditions under which food was sold in the 'market places'. In some areas, the stalls were not that far from the litter, making it possible for the flies to commute between the food tables and the rubbish dumps. This was particularly dangerous if the food sold was already cooked. There are many areas in other parts of the country where this is the case. In the Pinetown area in KwaZulu-Natal I accompanied women who cooked food in their homes and sold it to workers in various firms. The women set their stalls under bushes, so close to the litter heaps that some men were sitting on rubbish dumps whilst eating their meal. The owners of firms do not let them use their grounds which would provide a slightly better environment for selling food.

Food availability and its hygienic storage and distribution was one of the issues which concerned and motivated Dr. Nta to build a bakery to provide fresh bread for the community. However, before building it he sent questionnaires not only to tuck shop owners but to their customers to find out if they would like a bakery in the area and if so, what would they want to see provided. The response was very positive and on the basis of the answers Dr. Nta built the bakery. I met him when the questionnaires were being returned and six months later the bakery was up and running. The ultimate aim was to make the bakery a co-operative within which tuck shop owners were to become shareholders to ensure the success of the bakery without putting the tuck shop owners out of business. The bakery is near Orange Farm. Even the tuck shops which are furthest from it find it nearer than going to town for their supplies.

Lack of health facilities in Orange Farm was a well acknowledged fact. Why were so few GPs in the area?:

> Well, the first reason is that the place is not safe, so doctors are not keen to take the risk of having their cars stolen or their surgeries broken into. But I also think that the main reason is financial. A lot of us earn our money from private patients who have medical aids. Few people who live in Orange Farm fall into this category since the availability of the scheme is dependent on the employment status of individuals. The high level of unemployment makes the area unattractive to many doctors. But I intend to build my next surgery in the centre of Orange Farm (Dr. Nta, 1997).

If these factors were barriers to his colleagues, how was he going to overcome them? Dr. Nta believed that few places are totally safe. It was for this reason that he had in his surgery a resident caretaker. As far as the finance was concerned, he agreed that doctors do need to earn a living and were therefore justified to locate where well-paying patients lived. However, he felt that profit from those locations could be used to set up services in other areas where people needed them even if they were not money spinning areas:

> There is no other way if we are serious about providing services to our communities. Those of us who, for whatever reason, are able to accumulate some profit from our earlier efforts, must think about medically deprived communities in our areas before we think of buying a Mercedes Benz. I am not saying that people must never buy cars they

want. I am simply posing a question of commitment, priorities and patience for things that one wants to achieve (Dr. Nta, 1997).

In my discussion with Dr. Nta, a number of things that he wanted to achieve emerged. One was to purchase equipment for the surgery which would improve the services to his patients. Many patients who came to the surgery would benefit if there was an X-Ray machine, for example:

> This is particularly the case in winter when patients go down with chest infections. You may suspect that they may be having pneumonia, but because you are not sure, you start them with a cheap first line drug. They come back, say after four days and they have not improved. You then move to the second line drug. It is only when they come back the third time that you put them on the third line drug. By this time the patient's condition has deteriorated with a possible admission to hospital. An X-Ray would tell you immediately if the patient has pneumonia and you can then start with the third line drug as soon as possible. But we do not just need a chest X-Ray machine, but one that can be used for different parts of the body (Dr. Nta, 1997).

Such an X-Ray machine would also be very useful in detecting fractures, some of which can be managed in the surgery by applying slings or plaster of paris. Those with complicated fractures could be sent to hospital with little delay thus preventing further complications. Dr. Nta felt so strongly about this that he wrote to all GPs in the area asking them to club together and buy the machines which they could use collectively for their patients:

> None of them wanted to know. I am stuck at the moment because I do not have enough money to buy the machine, but it is a priority on my agenda as soon as I finish paying the bond (mortgage) on the second surgery (Dr. Nta, 1997).

The other two pieces of equipment that Dr. Nta thought would be useful were a scanner and an ECG machine. The advantage of these was that a hospital consultant could be presented with the results of the investigation when a patient was referred which meant that treatment could be started straight away instead of waiting for months to have an examination.

The other long term objective for Dr. Nta was to establish a comprehensive health centre which would serve not only the immediate areas of Orange Farm, Palm Springs and Lakeside, but also the big nearby township of Sebokeng whose hospital was in danger of closing down because of poor provision and lack of medical personnel. In his surgery he already had health workers who came in on specified days to provide their respective services. In a health centre, the number of such professionals would be greatly increased and the services provided wide-ranging. Dr. Nta was clear that the planning of such a Centre would need to balance long term survival strategies with the ability to provide services to those who may not be able to pay for them.

Dr. Nta identified a number of things from which he believed his patients would benefit. Did his patients share his views? He did not know because he had not asked them. Did he think it would be a good idea to ask them?

It is the obvious way forward, I just had not thought about it.

Why not? He did consult people before setting up a bakery, why not ask the patients about their health needs? He admitted that it could be the familiar scenario of a doctor-patient relationship in which 'doctor knows best'.

Once we agreed that the views of the users should be sought, we discussed what format the consultation should take. We opted for a focus group model which drew from the 'Open Space' approach introduced by Harrison (1993) and the INFRALAB experiment associated with Van Zuylen (1995) in Holland.

The success of the 'Open Space' approach, suggests Harrison, lies in the passion which participants bring to the discussion and the willingness to take personal responsibility to make things happen:

> Once the participants have gathered in a circle, they are invited to identify any issue or opportunity dealing with the theme at hand, for which they have some real passion and are willing to take personal responsibility. The requirement for passion differentiates Open Space from a variety of brainstorming techniques which often produce good ideas for somebody else to do. The requirement for the responsibility makes it quite clear that the 'somebody' is the proposer and it is the proposer's responsibility to convene the discussion on the item. When passion and responsibility are linked, effective action is a usual consequence. At the very least passion and responsibility provide the motive power for the Open Space event. (Harrison, 1993)

The INFRALAB experiment stresses the need to involve participants at every level in the development of a service: identifying a need, finding a solution and enacting the plan. An agreed priority list drawn from participants' contribution is sent out in the form of a questionnaire to a larger sample in the community to check if the list represents the views of other people. Both models stress that the very act of bringing people together to share views on issues is a very crucial part in the problem solving process. Some solutions do not need extra resources but a different way of perceiving and doing things.

The Consultation Process

What we did not have in this programme were resources in terms of time and personnel to advertise the meeting widely. We had two weeks during which patients who came to the surgery were informed about the meeting. In addition Dr. Nta contacted community groups and professionals working in the locality in order to get a wider view of what people perceive health needs to be. A total of 23 people came to the meeting, 17 women and six men. There was only one professional, a nurse from one of the clinics. Considering that this was on a Sunday afternoon, it was indeed a good turnout for people who were not familiar with such meetings. Dr. Nta, who has an affable personality further relaxed the atmosphere by providing drinks, biscuits and crisps. He led the session and opened with 'what can we do to ensure that we have good health and effective health services'. Even though I had been introduced as a researcher at the beginning of the discussion, people did not say things for the benefit of the researcher. They discussed issues about which they felt very strongly and they welcomed the opportunity to share these problems with each other. Dr. Nta used a flip chart to record all contributions.

Results of the Consultation

In presenting the results of the workshop I will start with the list of themes that were recorded on the flip charts as they were put forward by the participants. This will be followed by another list which emerged as the group agreed to priorities.

Tarring of the Roads There were no tarred roads in the area and when it rained the dirt roads became muddy and children who walked through them on their way to and from school invariably got dirty. The roads were covered with water after the rains because the drainage system is poor. The sewerage pipes were superficially laid and got easily damaged.

Need for a Clinic Many people in the meeting felt disadvantaged by the fact that there was no clinic in their vicinity. All state clinics provided free primary health care. Lack of such a facility in the area meant that people had to use GP services and these were too expensive for some people. Participants were angered by the decision taken by the government to shelve the building of a public clinic in this area. At this discussion it was agreed that the group should form itself into a committee and begin to challenge the decision.

Ambulance Facilities There were very few ambulances in the area. When called, they took a long time to come and they did not have life saving facilities in them. Some of them were just 'shells with not even a drip in them'.

Refuse Facilities The refuse service was very poor. Every Friday people were supposed to put their household refuse in a bin bag and place it in a big bin at the corner of their streets. But the bin collectors did not go to every street. The result was that the bin bags eventually spilt their contents and people became discouraged and simply threw their rubbish anywhere. A lot of dirt collected on the streets and in areas where children played. Flies commuted between these dirt heaps and houses. The issue about refuse collection and the tarring of roads was more than simply a system being inefficient. It was linked to the non-payment of rates and rent and the council's determination to restrict services in order to force people to pay. Some areas went for hours and sometimes for days without water. This was seen as unfair since in those areas some people were paying for services and were up to date with the rents.

Crime There was a concern about the high crime rate in the area. The police station was far away and by the time police came, the criminals had fled the scene. Besides, many people had no phones in their homes and public ones were, more often than not, vandalised. The suggestion was to have a police station in the area.

The Presence of Non-violent Thieves This was put forward as a warning about people who knocked on doors selling furniture polish or air freshener sprays. Into the containers, the thieves added an ingredient which produced deep sleep, thus making it easy for them to re-enter the house and take what they want, as one participant stated:

They work on the principle that women like to try out what they have bought immediately. So the thieves usually come in the afternoon when they know most women are at home on their own and doors are not usually locked as they are at night (Participant, 1997).

Condition of Schools Some school grounds were dirty and many school buildings had broken windows. There was a suggestion that people who lived near schools should remain vigilant in order to reduce vandalism. In many schools, toilets did not work and even in those areas where they did work, they were dirty and unhygienic. Although teachers were invited, none of them were at the meeting. It was agreed that they should be contacted to look at this issue and be invited again for the next meeting.

Health Education There was a need for extensive health education in order to enable people to take responsibility for their own health. People were encouraged to get in touch with the Department of Health and get leaflets on what was available and how to access it. The nurse who raised the point explained that such leaflets gave information on topics such as malnutrition, breastfeeding, TB, Hypertension, Diabetes and AIDS, areas in which user participation is crucial in minimising the impact on the health status of individuals and communities.

A Need for More Meetings As people became more involved in the discussion there was a call for more meetings which would bring people together to look at issues. Such meetings should be widely advertised and all stakeholders should be invited. People must be made aware of existing structures. The aim should not be to duplicate them but to get involved to ensure that they work effectively. It should be made clear that in these meetings there are no political allegiances. People must come together as concerned citizens to look at their needs.

A Need for a 24 Hour Service There were no emergency services in the area. People wanted nurses who could prescribe drugs to be in the surgery when the doctors were off duty.

A Need for Community Buildings A number of functions were put forward for such buildings - worship, community meetings, health workshops, youth clubs and conferences.

Recreation Facilities There were some open spaces in the area and people wanted these to be used for developing parks with trees which would improve the environment of the area. They wanted them to include areas for children's playgrounds with all the facilities to enhance child development.

Violence in Schools Almost all schools were facing violence from pupils attending them. The situation was terrifying to both teachers and pupils to an extent that teachers were going to school with guns for protection. Participants felt that they, as community members, must organise themselves into security groups who would be able to take guns away and to search all children for dangerous weapons. If any were found, they would be confiscated and parents informed. This should be accompanied by disciplinary measures.

The Role of Parents There was a lot of stress on the role parents play in the elimination of violence. At an early age, parents should teach their children what is bad and good behaviour. If children were brought up in this way, then they would be more likely to follow the guiding principles whether parents were there or not. When children get involved in criminal/delinquent behaviour, parents should not protect them by denying their children's involvement in such behaviour.

When people felt they had said all they wanted to say, we moved to the second phase of this consultation process - prioritisation.

Clinic/Health Centre People wanted a comprehensive health service. It did not matter what it was called so long as it had the following provisions:
- doctors/nurses;
- examination equipment - X-Ray scanner and ECG machines;
- 24 hour service for emergencies;
- ante natal and post natal care;
- delivery beds;
- recovery rooms where people can rest if they are quite ill;
- minor injury services and dressing of wounds;
- the availability of other health or health related professionals;
- availability of a room or shelter to be used for immunisation. At the time, parents waited for ages in the rain or heat at mobile clinic points.

Ambulance Service People were recounting examples when they had witnessed people dying of injuries whilst waiting for an ambulance which took ages to come. Similarly people with acute attacks of angina, asthma or diabetes had been left for a long time waiting for the ambulance service. Some believed that people's lives could have been saved if the ambulance had been available to take them to hospital.

The Establishment of a Police Station This was suggested as a third priority. This proposition was partially supported. Everyone agreed that dealing with crime and violence was indeed a priority. However, for a number of reasons, the police were not seen as the appropriate agents for this. Firstly, people felt that they should build their own communities and sort out issues for themselves. Secondly, they wanted to take responsibility for one another and whilst doing that, they did not want to be monitored by the police. Thirdly, and more importantly, historically police as agents of the apartheid regime, destroyed communities and people still carry physical and psychological scars. As a result, people have little trust or confidence in the police force. Fourthly, people would probably not commit crimes if police were around but that was seen as external control. What people wanted was to develop a sense of self-worth and respect for others, whether or not the police were there. It was that respect which stopped people from committing crime. Finally, people drew from their own experiences and concluded that even when the police were called, when they did come they did nothing. Although having a police station was not eventually seen as a priority, people felt that the chairperson of the police forum should be invited for the next meeting to explore how relations between the community and the police could be improved. People wanted to know what they could do to support the community police forum.

Health Education Health education was seen as a powerful tool since it had the potential to empower people by imparting knowledge which would enable them to be effectively involved in their own health needs. Another plus for health education was that it could be done with minimum resources. Classes or seminars on breastfeeding, immunisation, the role of vegetable gardens in the eradication of malnutrition, AIDS, sexually transmitted diseases and many more could be held in existing school halls at no cost at all since health educators would do it as part of their on-going work.

Removal of Refuse A committee was to be formed from this group to approach the council to do something about the rubbish on the streets, drainage pipes and the interrupted water supply.

Discussion

The prioritisation process was cut short as people wanted to get home before dark. We anticipated this since we only had an afternoon. Dr. Nta explained his own concern about lack of examination equipment in his surgery and assured the group that he would make this his priority. It would take time because of financial constraints but he had no doubt that such services would be made available. He made a similar commitment in relation to a health centre but this would be long term since he wanted to establish a surgery in the informal settlement of Orange Farm first. The establishment of the health centre, he stressed, must be a community effort:

> I am aware of the short fall in what we provide in our surgery. But we need to hear from you about what you need before we make our decisions. You must tell us what you are not happy about. It has been good that we met today. We need to continue the process. We have just recruited a second doctor into the practice and very soon we will be getting a third one. That means we will be able to provide the 24 hour cover that you suggest. As far as the health centre, the ambulance and the immunisation shelter are concerned, this will have to be a team effort. We all have to think about sources of funding. We should be able to mobilise the business community and other community groups to contribute financially for the shelter, for example. At the same time we must talk to nurses and suggest the use of such a shelter if it were to be available. The same approach must be adopted in relation to the ambulance and the health centre. We must all think of ways of raising funds. We cannot just sit and wait for the government to do it all (Dr. Nta, 1997).

Although the prioritisation process was cut short, enough was said to confirm that the need for equipment was not just Dr. Nta's perception, even though that perception on its own would be valid because, as a doctor, he had an overall picture and was aware of the impact lack of equipment had on his patients. It was reassuring to find that the users also identified the same need.

An important feature of action research is the production of interim/progress reports, verbal or written, rather than waiting for the final report at the end of the research. The aim here is to provide an opportunity for some action/intervention in response to some uncovered needs during the research process. Such interventions do re-assure people that the research is not just an academic exercise. In that context a report on the results of the group consultation was presented to the commissioner with a suggestion that there might be appropriate areas to which contribution could be made in order to meet some identified needs. The response of the commissioner was positive. Enough money was found to pay for a sonar, ECG and X-Ray machines.

From an action research perspective this was a successful research exercise which incorporated a number of major stages in the research process. A need for equipment was identified by Dr Nta, the provider. The views of the users were sought through a consultation process. Users identified a similar need. The information was passed on to the commissioner who provided funding to meet the identified need. Eleven months after installation of the equipment a quick evaluation was undertaken and the figures below confirm that a need was being met.

Table 11.1 Number of patients who have used equipment in Dr. Nta's surgery

X-Ray	327
Sonar	123
ECG	67

Another positive result of this study was the formation of the committee which campaigned for the establishment of a public clinic. The group was successful. Funds were made available by the government in South Africa to build the clinic. The committee was involved at every level of development. The clinic was officially opened in April 1998.

References

Harrison, O. (1993), *Open Space Technology: A User's Guide*, Abbott Publishing, Potomac, Maryland, U.S.A.

Van Zuylen, H.J. (1995), *Planning: The Creation of a New Reality*, Dutch Ministry of Transport, Public Works and Water Management, Transport Research Centre, Holland.

12 Quantitative Research

In this research a variety of methods have been used in collecting information on the health needs of black people in South Africa. The most dominant has been the qualitative in its broadest sense. Apart from the familiar planned in-depth interview technique, this has involved engaging people in conversation at every opportunity irrespective of time, place or situation. What I learnt from this approach is that what people say in a casual conversation is a far richer source of information on a whole range of experiences than I could get from organised interview approaches. My very first interview was a casual conversation with a young woman I met on a train on my second day in South Africa.

Thandi was on her way to work and had taken a train from Khayelisha (a black township) to Kenilworth (a white suburb) to see her sister who worked there as a domestic servant. In the conversation she told me that she and her sister came from Hanover, a rural area where they lived with their elderly parents who relied on them for a living. Wages in their hometown were very low, R100 a month, so they decided to move to Cape Town. She found a part time job cleaning an office for which she was paid R50 per half day. Thandi and her sister had a house in Khayelisha, in B side. At that stage my knowledge of informal settlements was fairly limited, so I asked for explanations:

What does B side mean?

It is a place where we put up our own homes using cardboard and whatever else we can find.

But don't they get soaked when it rains?

No, not all the time because we use the shiny stuff to close the holes in the cardboard. It is only when it rains heavily that we have problems with rain getting in the house. What is a real problem when it happens is fire. Because the shacks are so close to each other, when one catches fire, then a lot more also get burned down. At one stage ten shacks were burnt down and many people were left with no homes.

203

What about security, how do you protect your homes from burglary?

Well we do lock them, but it is easy to break into a cardboard house. But in general people do not steal because if they are found out, and they do get found out, they just get beaten up by other people in the area. Everybody knows that, so very few people will take a chance on stealing.

What about your health, does living in a cardboard house not affect your health?

Oh it is alright, we are not ill.

Does that mean you do not need anything done to improve your health?

Well we do need toilets, we do not have any on B side.

So how do you manage?

We go and ask people with toilets in their houses. When we first came we used to go to the police station and use outside toilets. But then they started locking them up so that we could not use them. We then found out that we could ask people to use their toilets.

What about water?

There are no water taps on B side, so we go with our buckets and get water from taps in people's yards. The people do not object because they know that there is no water on B side.

I presumed at the time that the people who offered their toilets and water must have been very understanding and sympathetic. It was not until I visited the townships that I discovered that these offers were made by house owners who were charging R50 per month per shack put up on their yards. In some areas the original four-roomed houses were barely visible in the midst of cardboard shacks.

Thandi was attending night school and she wanted to go to university but she thought it would be too expensive. She and her sister came to work in order to support their family back home. They were the younger members of an extended family for whom they had responsibility. The thought of using her earnings for university was totally out of question.

In that twenty minute conversation, a number of social factors which impact on health were indicated - employment, education, housing, sanitation, water, safety and crime. It effectively mapped out important areas to consider in assessing the health needs of black people in South Africa. The same areas came up time and time again in the course of subsequent conversations and planned in-depth interviews with individuals and focus groups.

Whilst I feel comfortable with the various aspects of the qualitative method, I do believe that there is an important role for quantitative data. Unlike Collinson, my conviction is not born out of the need to convince the 'Establishment' which has preference for the 'respectable' questionnaire surveys (Chambers, 1994). I think it is important to get the general picture, particularly if the aim is not just to gather information, but is to provide a service. This needs a larger sample than that offered by the qualitative method so that as many people as possible can have an in-put in determining which services are given priority. Fortunately, this general picture is already known in South Africa as a result of a number of research projects conducted within the country.

The National Household Survey of Health Needs (Hirschwitz and Orkin, 1995) collected information from 400 Africans, 150 coloureds, 100 Indians and 150 whites throughout the country in metropolitan areas, smaller urban centres, informal settlements and rural areas. The research was commissioned by NPPCHN as part of their campaign to put health on the agenda. The information accessed was biographical, demographic, attitudinal and experiential. It covered maternal and child health, sexual health, affordability and future expectations. The general picture from the survey showed Africans to be the most disadvantaged at both macro and micro levels of health. The results on education, employment, water and sanitation were echoed in my conversation with Thandi, and the rest of the people interviewed using the qualitative methods. There was no need therefore to pursue a similar questionnaire survey to cover the same areas. Our quantitative method was specifically concerned with checking if the information collected from our 'living with people' approach, casual conversations, in-depth interviews and focus groups was shared by a larger sample. The questions in the questionnaire reflected what people identified as their needs rather than the researcher deciding that these were the important questions to ask. Not only were questions asked, but in some instances the respondents were asked to prioritise the needs from their own perspective.

Quantitative data was collected from two settings - urban and rural. The urban study covered two areas, one in Gauteng and the other in KwaZulu-Natal. The two urban areas had the same questionnaire whereas the rural one drew questions from themes that were raised by women in in-depth interviews based on their experiences.

Methodology

Discussing the origin of Rapid Rural Appraisal (RRA), Chambers suggests that the main factors that led to the emergence of RRA, an approach which uses flexible methods such as 'opportunism, improvisation, iteration and cross-checking', are disillusionment with normal processes of questionnaire surveys and their results and the attraction of adaptability with no blue print program in the process of collecting information:

> Again and again, over many years and many places, the experience has been that large scale surveys with long questionnaires tended to be drawn out, tedious, a headache to administer, a nightmare to process and write up, inaccurate and unreliable in data obtained, leading to reports, if any, which were long, late, boring, misleading, difficult to use, and anyway ignored (Chambers, p.969).

In this study a number of factors made it particularly important to take note of Chambers' advice not to follow a blue print laid down by the traditional protocols, but to be flexible and adaptive in using the questionnaire method in order to meet the needs of the study and the imperatives of the local situation. Firstly, the questionnaire had to be short. It would have been inadvisable to produce a long drawn out questionnaire for people who are not familiar with form filling and whose priorities and time revolve around issues of survival and how to make ends meet. Secondly, it is known that when questionnaires are administered by a researcher going from door to door, the response rate is higher than when interviewees are left to fill-in and return the forms. In this study it was not easy for me to engage in a door to door exercise. I had limited time to spend in any one area, I was not familiar with the area and more importantly, as many people pointed out, it was not safe. There is still a lot of violence in South Africa and when one is not familiar with the set up, one becomes more vulnerable. That situation had implications for the drawing out of a sample and the decision about where questionnaires were to be distributed.

Sampling

Random sampling is the most favoured in survey-based research because of its ability to provide a reasonably representative sample. For a satisfactory random sampling it is essential that there is maximum access to the community within which the sample is drawn. For the reasons stated above, this was not possible in this study. However, since the objective was to elicit information from people who use the service, it felt appropriate to take a sample from the people who were visiting their general practitioner. To make the task easy for the surgery staff who were helping with the distribution of the questionnaires, the sampling was in time block. All patients who visited Dr Nta's surgery in a specified period of one month were given a questionnaire and asked to return it when filled. Two hundred questionnaires were given out. The overall response was poor with only 51 questionnaires returned. It could be that people were not interested in filling in the forms, or they had literacy problems. Either way, the poor response was important in informing the direction to take when conducting the same survey in KwaZulu-Natal.

In KwaZulu-Natal a surgery was again identified, but instead of giving the questionnaires out a research assistant interviewed patients as they were waiting to be seen or after the doctor had seen them. The relative safety of the area encouraged the assistant to venture outside the surgery and interview people waiting for their pension. The response was good. Out of 200 questionnaires, 170 were filled. Amongst those who declined to take part were men who wanted payment or to be given a qualification for filling in the form. Some were in a rush after having been seen by the doctor and others said they saw no point in filling these forms since everyone knows what is needed.

Results of the Questionnaires

The combined Gauteng and KwaZulu-Natal response was 221 - 23 percent from the Gauteng study and 77 percent from the KwaZulu-Natal study.

Since the sample was taken from people at the point of visiting their GP, we anticipated that the majority of the respondents would be women because, for a variety of reasons discussed elsewhere, more women tend to visit their GPs than men (Torkington, 1994). This was borne out in the results - 54 percent were women, 44 percent were men and two percent did not give their sex.

Because of the inclusion of pensioners, and the fact that younger people are relatively healthier and do not visit their GPs as often as older people, we expected a higher representation of people above 35 years. That expectation, as the chart shows, was also borne out in the results.

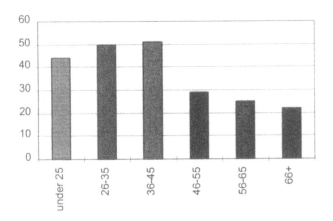

Figure 12.1 Age of respondents

Although a number of questions were asked to get the general picture, the main focus was on specific areas that had been mentioned in the focus groups and individual interviews. The group in Dr Nta's surgery had mentioned that one piece of equipment they wanted was an X-Ray. In this study respondents were asked to list services available in their doctors' surgeries. Only 8.6 percent mentioned that X-Ray machines were available. When people were asked what other services they thought should be available in the surgery, 41 percent mentioned an X-Ray. When asked what services were available in their local clinic, 31 percent mentioned an X-Ray, 69 percent did not. This is more worrying because a doctor would normally refer people to a clinic for X-Ray. If clinics have no machines, patients have to go to hospitals, miles from where they live.

One of the concerns that people expressed in the in-depth interviews was the length of time they had to wait before they were attended at the clinic. This varied from one hour to ten months with two people saying 'long enough' and 'too long'.

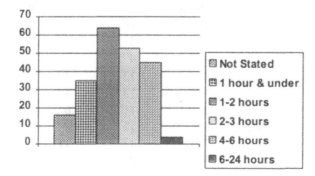

Figure 12.2 Length of time waited

It is possible for people to wait for two or three days before they are seen. Some clinics adhere to their closing time irrespective of whether or not there are still patients to be seen. There is no appointment system or any mechanism to ensure that people who are not seen the day before are given priority the following day. This was a real problem for people who had far to travel. Sometimes people gave up and did not come back until the condition became worse when they again made an effort to visit the clinic. This explains why some people put ten months, long enough and too long.

From focus groups and individual interviews a number of services that people felt were necessary for good health were identified. These services were compiled into a list and respondents were asked to indicate which of these were the most important by numbering them from 1-18, starting with the most important. In the overall sample the first five services were, ambulance, clinics, housing, sanitation and recreational facilities. For the two areas, however, differences in ranking emerged with the exception of housing which was ranked at four by both. For the KwaZulu-Natal sample the first five were: ambulance, effective sanitation, recreational activities, housing and clinics. For the Gauteng sample they were employment, clinics, prevention of crime, housing and ambulance.

Table 12.1 Priorities in health needs

	KwaZulu /Natal	Gauteng	Overall Sample
Halls for Community Gatherings	11	18	12
Crime Prevention	9	3	7
Housing	4	4	3
Effective Sanitation	2	13	4
Recreational Activities	3	12	5
Health Education	6	7	6
Elimination of School Vandalism	8	15	9
Tarring of Roads	7	17	11
Clinics	5	2	2
Police Station	10	6	8
Employment	12	1	10
Removal of Refuse	13	8	13
A feeding scheme for malnourished children	15	9	14
Services for terminally ill people.	16	14	16
Counselling for people with AIDS and cancer	17	10	17
Drop in centre for rape victims and their families	18	11	18
Crèche	14	16	15
Ambulance	1	5	1

Discussion

Although the sample is small and therefore it would be regarded as insufficient for generalisation, it is important to remember that the themes originated from a variety of people in different settings in the three provinces where this research was conducted. The main role of the sample is not to establish facts but to cross check what has already been identified by using other methods. In terms of generalisation it should not be assessed as an independent method but as part of the triangulation process.

Despite its size, a number of interesting points have emerged. It has identified similarities and differences in the two provinces in what people regard as important for good health. It has shown that people have a very strong macro conception of health. At a micro level, people are very clear about what should be available in doctors' surgeries and clinics.

The macro conception of health is reflected in the average ranking of housing, sanitation and recreation within the first five services regarded important for health. The awareness of the importance of the role of these social factors, however, has not detracted focus on health needs at a micro level as indicated by the allocation of ambulance and clinic at one and two respectively. Differences, however, begin to emerge when we look at the individual province ranking. Whilst the total ranking represents the overall-need picture the individual ranking reflects local history and experiences. In the Gauteng sample, for example, the first five are employment, clinics, crime prevention, housing and ambulance service. For the KwaZulu-Natal sample priorities are ambulance, effective sanitation, recreation, housing and clinics.

It is not surprising that the first concern for the Gauteng sample is employment. The area is far from the city and has a poor transport service. It is not easy to travel to Gauteng (Johannesburg) or Verenniging to look for work. Even if people were to get employment in these cities, their wages would be eroded by taxi fares. For these reasons, people need employment in areas in which they live. There are very few clinics available in Orange Farm and the neighbouring townships of Palm Springs, Lakeside, Evaton and Seboking in relation to the size of the population. At the time of the study there was no clinic serving the residents of the townships near Orange Farm, hence the need for clinics was ranked second. Gauteng and its townships and peri-urban areas have the highest record on crime in the country and in the world. It was not surprising therefore that the prevention of crime was given priority. Housing was rated equally in the two provinces. The need for the ambulance, ranked at five, may suggest that the overall health provision is so poor that the availability of the ambulance was not seen as that important if in fact the clinics to which people were taken were not efficient in the treatment they provided. It could also be that the perception of ambulances is that they were no more than 'empty shells'.

Although Clermont, an area from which the KwaZulu-Natal sample was drawn, had some new people who had come as a result of political disturbances in the early and mid 1990s, the majority of people were residents who had lived there for generations. They had had good ambulance services until hijacking and the beating up of ambulance drivers became the norm. In the past doctors were able to call the ambulance with no difficulties. As one doctor pointed out, when the ambulance is now called the response is, 'sorry we can't come out because that will put our drivers in danger and we will also lose the ambulance'. The need for the ambulance therefore is felt far more sharply by people who have had a reasonable service in the past. The availability of clinics on the other hand is ranked at five which appears to suggest that people are generally happy about this provision. This may be so compared to what was available in the Orange Farm area, but the other possible explanation is that Clermont is near hospitals in the Durban area which may mean that people rely less on clinics than the people in Orange Farm. Although Clermont residents had been in the area for a long time, most of them built their own homes and the quality reflected the economic capacities of individual families. Some of the homes have lacked effective sanitation for many years, hence the ranking of this facility at two. By contrast, the part of Orange Farm that was adjacent to the surgery where the sample was drawn, had toilets that had been built through the RDF programme. Other respondents were from the townships that had water toilet systems, hence the ranking of sanitation at 13.

The Clermont community has had no recreational facilities for a long time and the previous government paid no attention to community representations for such facilities. People generally felt that the ANC government with its emphasis on provision for the young will be more responsive to the need of recreational facilities in the area.

The differences must not obscure the fact that the two areas put in their top five, three services: housing, clinics and ambulances. On that basis it is reasonable to conclude that these will be amongst the most needed facilities for good health in the country. But what is equally interesting in these findings is the low ranking given to services for people with AIDS and rape victims. Given that both these areas have a very high profile in the country, one would have expected them to rank high in the responses.

Similarly, lack of services for terminally ill people, crèche facilities and feeding schemes for malnourished children are not high in the ranking system. There are probably a number of reasons for this. One is that all of these areas tend to be seen in terms of individuals rather than the system and therefore have some degree of shame/guilt attached to them. Despite the economic difficulties that are outside the control of individual families, people still feel responsible if their children are not fed well. This is why women will juggle the little resources they have at their disposal, including starving themselves, to make sure that their children have something to eat. It is the same sense of responsibility and the fact that many mothers who do not work are at home and they therefore do not see an urgent need for crèche facilities. It is the same sense of responsibility, I would argue, which accounts for the low ranking of services for people who are terminally ill. People feel that it is their responsibility to look after their ill relatives. With AIDS and rape the factor of shame and lack of information are responsible for the low ranking. I have no doubt that increased health education, which is ranked at six by the Clermont respondents and at seven by the Orange Farm respondents, will sharpen people's understanding and make them realise that these are not just their own individual problems that they alone can solve. They are national problems and they need national solutions.

It was interesting to note that people's expectations from their GPs were not limited to equipment but to the doctor-patient relationship and the environment within which they were treated. Some people, for example, wanted to have more time with the doctor to discuss their illness and to talk in general about health. Others wanted to have a proper and clean waiting room. The GP system in South Africa appears to suit the patient in the sense that if people are not happy with a GP they can go to another one whenever they choose. In practice this is not as simple as it looks. Whilst some people in urban areas may have this opportunity, in general this is not possible because there are very few doctors available. There are even fewer doctors who provide what patients are looking for. The choice for many people is academic rather than practical especially in rural areas.

The Vulamehlo Study

The findings in this study are of particular interest to me. I was born and brought up in this area and whilst living in England, have made repeated return visits to my family. I have therefore experienced life here and have witnessed the changes as they have taken place on a year to year basis. Knowing the area and the people has given me some confidence in evaluating the accuracy of the responses to some questions in the questionnaire. This remains the case despite the fact that I have lived in England for many years where my perceptions, to some extent, have been influenced by my experiences in those years.

Methodology

The themes used to construct the questionnaire emerged from the in-depth interviews and the discussion groups held with different women in the course of the research process in the Vulamehlo area. Since in this area women were the most active in every aspect of life, and therefore the most affected by lack of health resources at both macro and micro levels, it made sense to restrict the sample to women. Two women were asked if they would be interested in acting as research assistants and administering questionnaires. The questionnaire, which was translated in Zulu, and the method of collecting information were discussed to ensure that the questions were asked appropriately and the answers recorded accurately.

In order to minimise literacy related difficulties in filling in the questionnaires, it was agreed that the interviewers would engage in a face to face interview and fill in the questionnaires. Women were interviewed in a variety of settings - in their homes, in the vegetable gardens and in group meetings. A total of 100 women were interviewed.

Results of the questionnaires

One area of concern which emerged in the in-depth interviews was the availability of fuel. To assess the extent to which this was a shared concern women were asked what fuel they used in cooking and lighting. For cooking 83 percent used firewood, 16 percent paraffin stove. For lighting 66 percent used candles, 34 percent paraffin lamp. None of the women used electricity for cooking or lighting. The concern in this area was around the difficulty in finding firewood and the expense of buying candles and paraffin.

In this area very few women were engaged in paid employment. This had an impact in their ability to provide for their families.

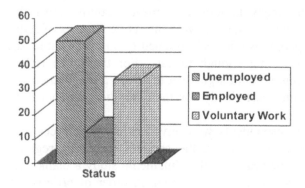

Figure 12.3 Employment status

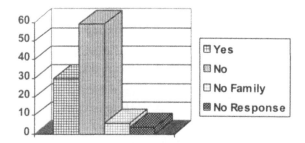

Figure 12.4 Ability to provide adequate subsistence for the family

It was quite interesting to note that 30 percent of the respondents said that they could provide for their families sufficiently. Given that only 13 percent of the women were employed, one wonders how so many could provide for their families sufficiently. The employing agency was the weaving centre which paid women according to their productivity. The highest paid received R200 a month. Even those whose husbands were employed in towns and cities, and there were not many, the wages they earned were not enough for sufficient provision. The majority of families do have fields from which they produce maize and beans, the latter in smaller amounts. Apart from women who cultivate vegetable gardens, sufficient food for many may mean maize prepared in different ways for breakfast, lunch and supper. Maize on its own has limited nutrients, in which case sufficient for many families may mean quantity rather than quality. Having lived in the area and knowing the subtle nuances of status, I also know that some people would feel ashamed to admit in public that their children were not having enough to eat. For them this reflects personal failure. From this I would argue that there are more women who find difficulty in providing sufficiently for their families than what the graph suggests.

In the urban surveys respondents were given a list of services from which to choose in order of priority, the services that they regarded important in improving their health. In the Vulamehlo study a blank sheet was given and women were asked to put down, in order of priority, the main things they felt would improve their life.

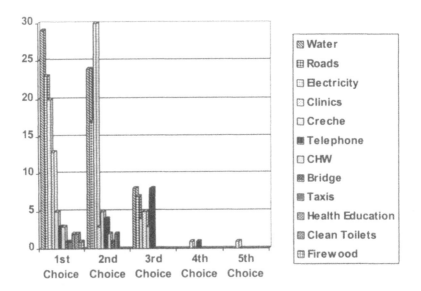

Figure 12.5 Things that would have a big impact on health (starting with the most important)

Water, electricity and roads featured as the most needed facilities in this area. These findings concur with the information which emerged from in-depth interviews. Women and young girls have the responsibility of fetching water. This is time consuming. Women are also aware that water from rivers is the source of many diseases, not least, the fatal cholera epidemics. It is not surprising therefore that women put this high on their list.

Alternative sources of fuel would have a liberating effect in terms of time spent in collecting firewood. Women still travel for miles to a white farmer's forest where they either pay or weed the farmer's field for a specified time before they can go and collect firewood. It is a whole day's work. They leave home at dawn and come back late afternoon carrying firewood on their heads. Other women, particularly elderly women who find it difficult to travel to the forest, use nearby natural scrub forests which will eventually be decimated because, unlike the farmer's forest, there is no replacement of what is cut down for fire. This has serious environmental consequences.

Lack of a good road system becomes a real problem when transport is needed to take an ill person to a clinic or hospital. It is not surprising that women identified the need for this service because they are the ones who take responsibility for ill members in their families.

In the in-depth interviews many women expressed their appreciation of the work of CHW in disseminating information about first aid treatment particularly with children. One area often mentioned was the treatment of diarrhoea.

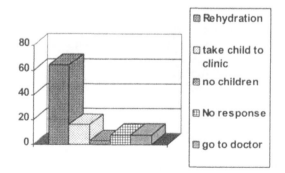

Figure 12.6 What do you do when your child has diarrhoea?

It was quite encouraging to note a change in the way women dealt with diarrhoea. In the past there was a shared belief that vomiting and diarrhoea were caused by deliberate poisoning by a witch doctor or his/her agent.

It was also believed that giving water to the patient would fuel the poison. For this reason water was not given no matter how much the patient begged for it. In those days I was not only the first person to train as a nurse in the area but I was also young and my newly gained knowledge about rehydration was dismissed as a dangerous childish prank. Only one woman who was desperate to save her baby boy was brave enough to try out what I was suggesting. I stayed the night with the family, not only to ensure that the fluid was administered regularly, but also to re-assure the mother that the baby was not poisoned and to explain why water was the only thing that had a chance to save her baby. Her doubt decreased as the baby's condition improved. The story of this first rehydration became legendary and the 'baby', who now has children of his own, still refers to me jokingly as 'my life saver'. As a result of the baby's recovery more women in the neighbourhood started giving water to their children when they had diarrhoea, but the practice was limited to our village. It is very encouraging indeed to find that 68 percent of the respondents use rehydration as the norm in the treatment of diarrhoea.

When women were asked where they took their children when ill, many (43 percent) did not give an answer to this question. Only seven mentioned traditional healers and one mentioned both traditional healers and clinic.

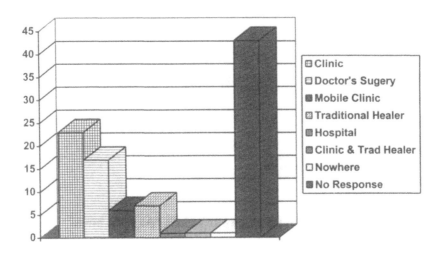

Figure 12.7 Where children are taken for medication when ill

I think the responses reflect lack of clarity in the question asked. The first line of treatment in this area is self-medication using local herbs. Depending on the nature of the illness most people, including children, recover during this initial treatment thus obviating the need for further treatment. Had the question been 'what do you do when your child is ill?' we would have had a different set of responses.

An interesting finding was in relation to CHW. Although 99 percent of respondents said that they would like to have CHWs in their area, only three people listed them as first priority and two as second priority. This reflects the dominance of curative medicine, traditional or Western, when people are ill. When CHWs' knowledge of traditional healing is widely acknowledged and promotional and preventative health care attains a higher profile, we may begin to see a different rating.

For the purposes of this research the survey method has been very useful in that it confirmed information collected through in-depth interviews, 'living with people' and focus groups.

References

Chambers, R. (1994), 'The Origins and Practices of Participating Rural Appraisal', *World Development*, vol.22, No.7.

Hirschwitz, R. and Orkin, M. (1995), *Hearing the People – A National Health Survey of Health*, NPPHCN, South Africa.

Torkington, N.P.K. (1994), 'Black Women and Health: A Political Overview of British Health Care', in Wilson, Melba, *Healthy and Wise*, Virago.

13 Action Research

The aim of this research was to look at the health needs of black people in South Africa in order that an area for intervention could be identified. The results of the survey, in-depth interviews and focus groups indicated that at a micro level ambulances and health centres, particularly for areas served by mobile clinics were the most urgently needed services. Some community groups were actively looking for funds to build their own centres. This provided an opportunity for appropriate intervention whereby assistance is given to community groups to meet their own identified needs. In response to the findings Jane, the commissioner of the research, set up a small trust, the Themba (Hope) Health Trust.

In the research respondents identified a whole range of areas in which services are needed – health and nutrition centre for under fives, services for elderly people, services for terminally ill people, health education, counselling, economic activities, literacy/numeracy and many more. It is unlikely for centres initiated by community groups which are aware of these needs to remain focussed only on curative services. Such centres are likely to be holistic and multi-purpose and therefore more able to provide other services which impact positively on health. Even if one community group has been enabled to meet its objective, the aim of action research to make a difference in people's lives shall have been fulfilled and more so if that one centre acted as a model and was replicated in other parts of the country. It is important, however, to acknowledge that tangible structures are not the only way in which research can make a difference in people's lives. During the research process there are opportunities for researchers to contribute to the empowerment of community groups with whom they interact. In this research an opportunity was taken to contribute to this empowerment process in a number of different ways.

Sharing Information

This study involved three provinces – Western Cape, KwaZulu-Natal and Gauteng. When people are involved in day to day activities, whether they be users or providers of services, they rarely have time to sit back and review what they are doing, never mind travel miles to see what other people do. This is not because they lack ability, it is because they lack time and resources to do so. As a researcher I had both. I had time to listen, ask questions and evaluate. On my travels between provinces I shared my understanding with other groups, not to impose ideas but to enable people to see how other areas dealt with similar problems. For example, I shared with other groups of providers and users information on the activities of the Philani Nutrition Health Centre in the Western Cape. The information was well received and some groups indicated that a nutrition centre will be considered in their future plans.

Another example relates to care for terminally ill people. In Cape Town I visited St Luke's Hospice and I was greatly impressed by the way the hospice service was not just promoted but was being taken to the homes of black people in the townships. I subsequently visited the Portshepstone Hospice in KwaZulu-Natal and the Houghton Hospice in Gauteng and compared the various ways each employed to reach the black community. I shared the information with people in Ndonyane, a rural area without such a service. We discussed with NGOs the possibility of linking up with the hospice covering the area so that terminally ill people could receive appropriate care in their homes and have access to hospitalisation when necessary.

The sharing of information was also useful at an individual level. People living in the area were not always aware of what was available. On many occasions I visited services and came back with information unknown to some people. A good example was the work of hospices. Many people to whom I spoke did not know of their existence and those who knew, did not know how they worked or how to access them. A similar lack of knowledge was evident in the area of alternative therapy. One woman in her 70s who has lived in the area all her life is now using steam treatment with a local alternative therapist as a result of this research:

> I have lived here all of my adult life and yet I have never heard of this therapist and he lives a mile from my house.

Listening to people

In some instances no information is needed from an outside agent. All one needs to do is listen and in listening one acknowledges the legitimacy of people's concerns and in that way gives them confidence to take appropriate steps to resolve their problems. This is exemplified in the case of a resident who took me to see her unfinished house built with the support of RDP funds. She was concerned that her two-roomed house had only one window. She felt that there was nothing she could do about it because no one would take notice of her complaint. I encouraged her to go and see her local councillor. She did and as a result the builders were told to put in a window in the other room. The success of this resident will have far-reaching rippling effects. She will share her positive experience with other people facing a similar situation who will be encouraged to challenge poor services. The councillor has been alerted to the poor quality of work and will be more vigilant in his monitoring. The builders know that people are not going to put up with shoddy work. These positive experiences increase people's confidence. They begin to feel empowered as they realise that the power to bring about change lies within them. Admittedly this will be a slow process punctuated by many failures but it is nevertheless a crucial way of bringing about a positive change in people's lives. When people begin to speak for themselves and start to exercise their rights, things begin to change.

Listening is not only essential when people talk about their problems but also when they talk about their success. In general people like to talk about their work. It is even more satisfying and encouraging to talk to an outsider who genuinely appreciates the work done and shares information about what is done in other parts of the country and in other countries. The outsider's appreciation does not just affirm the value people put on their work but it increases that value and this gives people confidence and inspiration to develop their potential. The sharing of information enables them to evaluate their own projects in comparison with what other people are doing elsewhere. This point was made very clearly by the Women's Voice of Orange Farm members who took me to their different projects:

> We like having visitors and showing them what we are doing here. We know we are doing important and good work for ourselves and our communities, but it is even nicer when people coming from outside say so as well. We also like sharing ideas and finding out what other people are doing and how we can improve on what we do.

Researchers are included in this process of affirmation. When people acknowledged my research as a useful undertaking it increased the value of what I was doing in my own eyes. It is in that mutual appreciation that participants find confidence and empowerment which propels them forward to new heights in whatever they are doing.

Creating Links Between Groups

When one works with different groups one gets to know their skills as well as their needs. This makes it possible to facilitate linkages between them. The Orange Farm experience provided an example of how this happened in this study. The women in Orange Farm had a variety of skills but they had a problem with literacy which is not resolved by the night school classes. When we discussed this literacy problem I mentioned to the women the existence of Women's Education for Southern Africa (WEFSA), a trust set up specifically to meet the literacy needs of women. I had already met the tutors whose main office was in Soweto and knew how their organisation worked. The women in Orange Farm welcomed the news and asked if I could facilitate a meeting between them and the tutors. The response from the tutors was quick, positive and enthusiastic. They accompanied me on visits to Orange Farm, not only to arrange literacy sessions with the women but to see their projects as well. One of the tutors had had lessons in brick making and she was very excited at the prospect of renewing and furthering her skills with the brick making group in Orange Farm. The same tutor has typing skills, an asset desperately needed by the Orange Farm group. Typing will now be part of the literacy package and this exchange of skills will create a healthy relationship of mutual benefit. Women in nearby townships heard about WEFSA and asked to have literacy in their areas.

Another link concerned sewing skills. On one of my visits to Orange Farm a woman from the sewing group brought in a finished skirt to be assessed for quality by the chairperson and other women in the office. Even I, with no sewing skills, could see that the finished product was of poor quality. I mentioned to the women the expertise of the Zamani Soweto Sisters and suggested a link with them. They are based in Soweto and take students to train in skills such as sewing.

In forging links it is important not to impose on groups. My role was to share information and when women expressed an interest link them with those who have the skills they need. Of equal importance is the fact that in all the above interactions, resources in the form of funding were not necessary and yet I believe the process was and remains crucial in unlocking the power within, which enables people individually or in groups to bring about lasting positive changes in their lives.

Conclusion

The end of the apartheid regime in 1994 left scars as evidenced in the quality of education, housing, welfare, employment and health services. Making these scars less invisible poses a major challenge for the ANC Government. The RDP sought to mobilise people and the country's resources toward the eradication of apartheid and its aftermath and the building of a democratic, non-racial and non-sexist future.

Crucially the house building project has provided many people with homes and some areas now have water supplies, toilets and electricity. The damage, however, has been so great and the inequalities so entrenched, that many initiatives have been dismissed as too little and ineffective. Others argue that the issue is not the amount of what is being done but the direction the government is taking to bring about transformation and its reluctance to tackle land redistribution which is central to the survival of millions of people in the rural areas. Most initiatives have favoured people in urban areas with an attractive infrastructure and job opportunities. But for those in the rural areas the only way to survive is to have productive land on which to grow food. Without the distribution of land South Africa is going to continue losing her children through malnutrition and related diseases. The urgency for land distribution was captured by Periman (1993):

> I hear talk of economic turnabout,
> of the miracle of foreign investment.
> But I see no benefit in this for the rural poor
> and I fear for the future of this land.
> I see a government that has no money
> to feed the newly hungry,
> But gives one million Rand to Malawi
> to create a reserve for two rhinos
> and I fear for the future of this land.
> When I see how carefully the talk shop at Kempton Park
> has avoided the issue of urgent land redistribution,
> which is the only hope of the functionally illiterate migrant
> who has been thrown out of work

> by the demise of many mines and by mechanisation in agriculture,
> and I know that 310 million acres (sic) of trust land are available now,
> then I fear for the future of this land.
> When I see that our three national imperatives,
> education, health and housing,
> have been referred to the new regions,
> and I think of the provincial and homeland track records,
> I fear for the future of this land.
> When I hear the above basic human rights
> called 'unreasonable expectations,'
> I fear for the future of this land.
> If the government of national unity,
> when it assumes power in 1994,
> does not have the giant courage to make immediate commitment
> to certain things, primarily to free and compulsory education
> and immediate and rapid land availability,
> then indeed I fear for the future of our land.
> (Periman, 1993, p.14)

It is against this wider backdrop of a society wounded by injustices of the past that I have looked at the health needs of black people. The themes identified expose shortfalls in health provision. Primary health care is available free to everyone yet lack of resources undermine it. Improvements in children's and women's health are compromised by the absence of national strategies to tackle malnutrition and combat violence.

Employment, the availability of land, particularly for those who cannot find employment, an effective welfare service, an effective judiciary system in South Africa have critical roles in attending to health needs and initiatives that enable people to regain their sense of humanity. It is through participation that our humanity is affirmed and it is in that affirmation that we may find confidence, trust, self-worth, self-love, self-respect and security. These elements contribute to what is known as 'ubuntu' in South Africa. A person with 'ubuntu' or a sense of being is less likely to engage in activities or lifestyles which are destructive to the self, others or the environment. It is people with 'ubuntu' who are also more likely to be receptive to Bhasin's suggestion:

> Wherever we are let us talk about and insist on values like justice, ethics, morality, beauty, love. Because these values were lost sight of, development lost its human face. We have to bring back these values into our private and public lives. Other values are reverence for all life, simple living, living in harmony with nature, respect for diversity.

Wherever we find there is no justice, morality, ethics, we have to speak up, not keep quiet. In the end I only want to say that large numbers of small groups all over the world are already doing what I have suggested here. Let us put in our bit to create a better world (Bhasin, 1992).

In making 'Herstory' women are engaging in that process of affirmation. The act of working as a group rather than competing with each other is a step in the right direction towards a search for that sense of being.

The slow progress in the democratisation process and the shortfalls in service provision must not obscure what has been achieved in a relatively short time. That people who have been brutally abused and dehumanised by the apartheid system have emerged with dignity to re-build their communities is a tremendous achievement. It was that dignity and the will to forgive and not avenge the injustices inflicted which enabled the Trust and Reconciliation Commission to function. The introduction of a free primary health care service is an attempt to ensure that health care is accessible and equitable to all irrespective of economic status. That there are still discrepencies should not eclipse the intention to have an equitable system of health care at this level. The development of garden projects, feeding schemes and increases in child allowance grant all hold much promise in the fight against child poverty and malnutrition which impact negatively on health. These factors acknowledge the wisdom in strengthening the fence at the top of the cliff rather than improving the ambulance service at the bottom of the cliff. In post apartheid South Africa surviving childhood is still an achievement for many black children.

Whilst the role of CHW is not generally recognised or nationally remunerated at present, it nonetheless holds much promise in the development of a comprehensive primary health care system. The promotion of CHW would be a great asset to many communities especially those in remote rural areas with poor health facilities.

The education programmes which are now available and accessible to adults in some parts of the country will have a tremendous impact in people's life chances and the extent to which they can engage meaningfully in the discussion of issues which affect their lives. Such programmes, however, need to go beyond literacy and numeracy skills and pay attention to other areas, e.g. nutrition, health, childcare, practical and employment skills, assertiveness, confidence building etc. Such a broad approach to education, particularly for women and mothers 'who hold up half the sky insofar as maintaining family life' (Bethlehem, 1997), would have a far reaching impact not only on health but on the overall development of families, communities and nation.

Enabling people to earn a living is another crucial way in which people's health and quality of life can be improved. Providing employment is one way of doing this. The other is the promotion of small businesses using the support of economic structures which makes it possible for people to borrow small amounts of money from banks. The Micro Credit Scheme initiated by Professor Muhammad Yunus (1998) in Bangladash works along these lines. The Grameen Bank lends money to borrowers who have no collateral. Such a scheme has enormous relevance to people in South Africa, not least because it has helped to lift a third (2.4 million) of borrowers from poverty.

Whatever is provided, education or service, it is absolutely crucial that this builds on existing local situations, knowledge expertise and practices. In general people know their locality better than professional providers. They know their own needs, understand local politics and tradition, they know what is culturally acceptable and what is not. They are therefore well placed to make suggestions on how information and services should be packaged in order to make them accessible and acceptable. This knowledge must be augmented and not replaced. It is important that the knowledge that local people have forms the basis for a genuine partnership within which their contribution is recognised, valued and acknowledged.

In the course of time people develop skills and expertise in response to their local needs. As these skills are passed on from generation to generation they become embedded and form part of traditional practice. The expertise of TBAs in Vulamehlo is a good example of a passed-on skill. The training the TBAs received from the Western-trained midwife built on existing traditional knowledge. Equality in partnership was enhanced by the exchange of information and the acknowledgement of good practices on either side. This did not only empower the women involved but it also affirmed the value of traditional knowledge. How we value people's knowledge and contributions is the acid test of whether or not we value their humanity.

It is my hope that this book will play a part in creating an environment in which we all value each others' contribution, knowledge and humanity.

References

Bethlehem, M. (1997), op. cit.
Bhasin, K. (1992), Unpublished Paper presented at the Fifth International Congress on Women's Health Issues in Copenhagen.
Caulkin, S. (1998), 'Credit Where Credit's Due', *Observer*, 15 November.
Periman, I. (1993), 'I Fear for the Future', in *Critical Health*, December, No.45.

For Product Safety Concerns and Information please contact our EU
representative GPSR@taylorandfrancis.com Taylor & Francis Verlag GmbH,
Kaufingerstraße 24, 80331 München, Germany

Printed and bound by CPI Group (UK) Ltd, Croydon, CR0 4YY
01/05/2025
01858511-0001